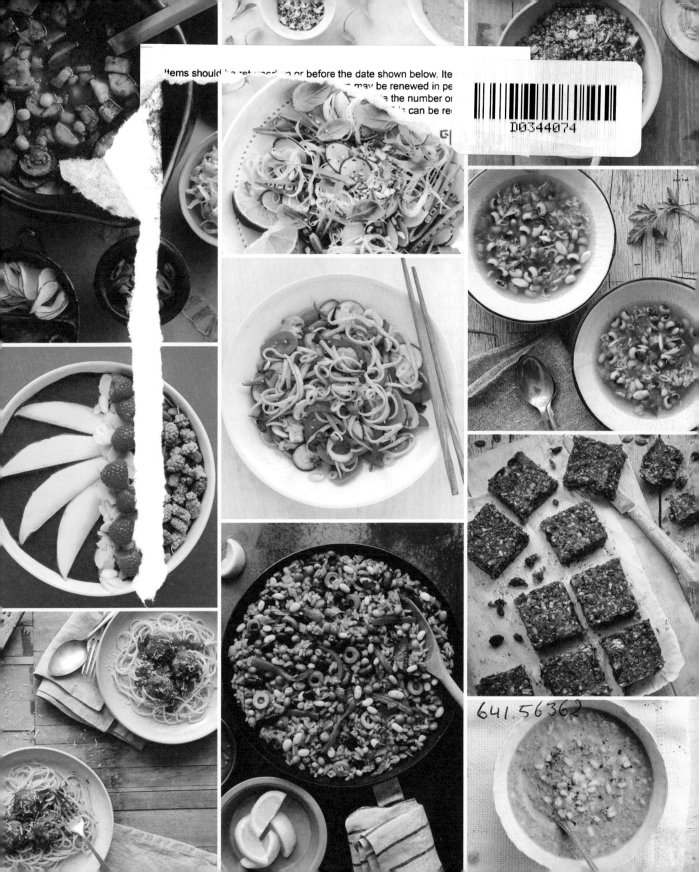

THERE'S A
VEGAN
IN THE HOUSE

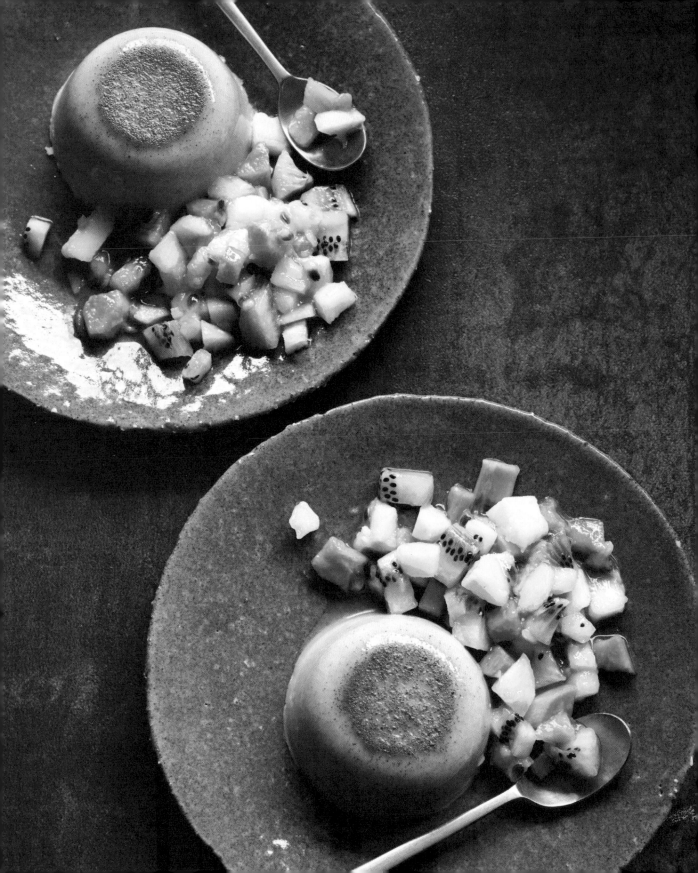

THERE'S A
VEGAN
IN THE HOUSE

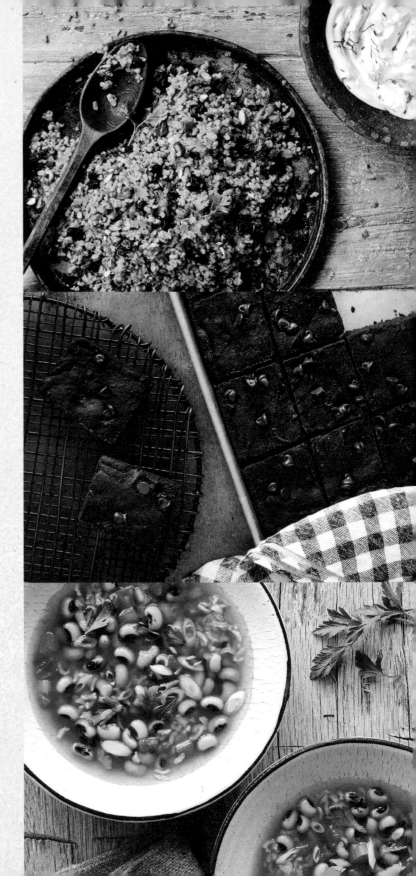

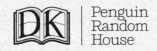

Consultant Heather Whinney
Editors Laura Bithell,
Anna Cheifetz, Helena Caldon,
Designers Steve Marsden,
Alison Gardner, Vanessa Hamilton
Jacket Designer Nicola Powling
Producer, Pre-production Heather Blagden
Producer Igrain Roberts
Indexer Michele Moody
Managing Editor Dawn Henderson
Managing Art Editor Alison Donovan
Art Director Maxine Pedliham
Publisher Mary-Clare Jerram

First published in Great Britain in 2019
by Dorling Kindersley Limited
80 Strand, London WC2R 0RL

Copyright © 2019 Dorling Kindersley Limited
A Penguin Random House Company
10 9 8 7 6 5 4 3 2 1
001 – 312714 – Jan/2019

All rights reserved.
No part of this publication may be reproduced,
stored in a retrieval system, or transmitted in any
form or by any means, electronic, mechanical,
photocopying, recording, or otherwise, without the
prior written permission of the copyright owner.

A CIP catalogue record for this book is available
from the British Library.
ISBN 978-0-2413-6284-6

Printed and bound in China

A WORLD OF IDEAS:
SEE ALL THERE IS TO KNOW

www.dk.com

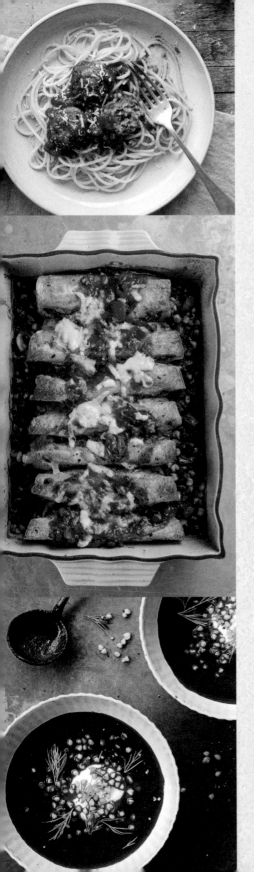

CONTENTS

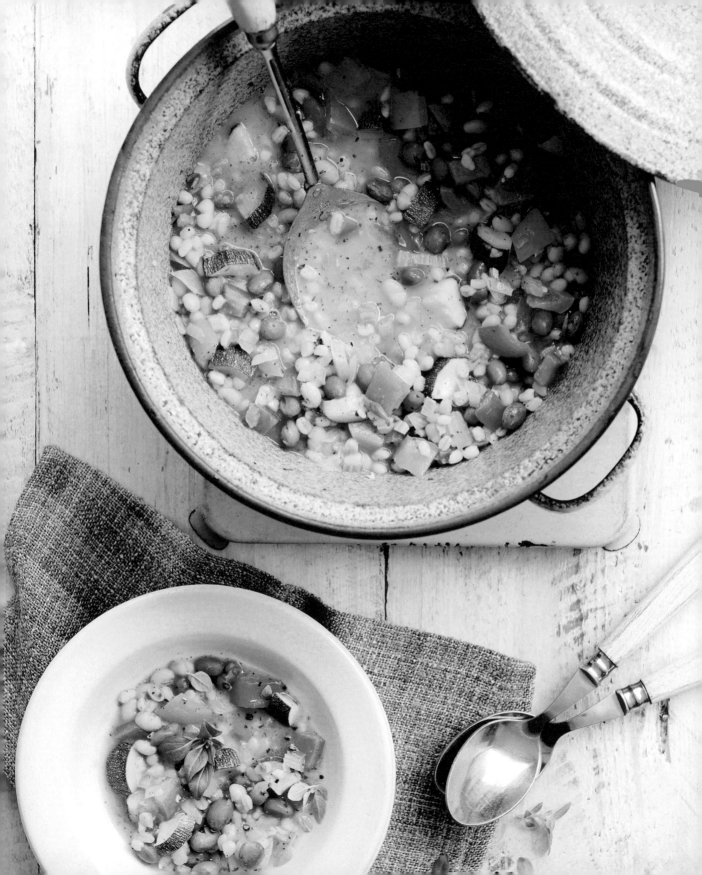

INTRODUCTION

It is increasingly common to live in a house in which at least one person is vegan. Veganism is steadily becoming one of the most popular diets worldwide, with people adopting a plant-based diet for reasons varying from environmental and animal welfare concerns to personal health. Vegans exclude all animal products from their diet – this includes meat, fish, eggs, and dairy, but also any product with an ingredient derived from animals. Some of these, such as certain brands of orange juice, may surprise you!

If you or a family member has decided to make the switch it's natural to have a few concerns. You may worry about maintaining a balanced diet or about finding somewhere to eat out. If it's your child who has decided to go vegan, perhaps you're worried they won't get enough calcium or iron. The introduction pages are written with this in mind – they tackle the myths of veganism, suggest the best animal product substitutes, advise on shopping and storing, and give you a full understanding of the nutrients the body needs and how to source these through a plant-based diet. "The good stuff" boxes on many recipes offer useful nutritional information and highlight the health benefits of each dish.

From hearty, healthy mains to delicious but not-so-naughty desserts, the 100-plus recipes in this book are designed to cover everyone's wants and needs. It is often easier to make the change to veganism gradually and not everyone in the household may be following the same diet. The "flex it" boxes are written for convenience and flexibility, so home-cooked meals can be eaten by vegetarians, pescatarians, meat-eaters, and flexitarians with just a few tweaks and additions to the recipes.

Eating a balanced diet is vitally important for all of us so a switch to veganism for one member of the household can be a good time to reconsider the whole family's eating habits. Discover the powerful potential of plant-based foods to take centre stage and to keep the whole household happy and well fed.

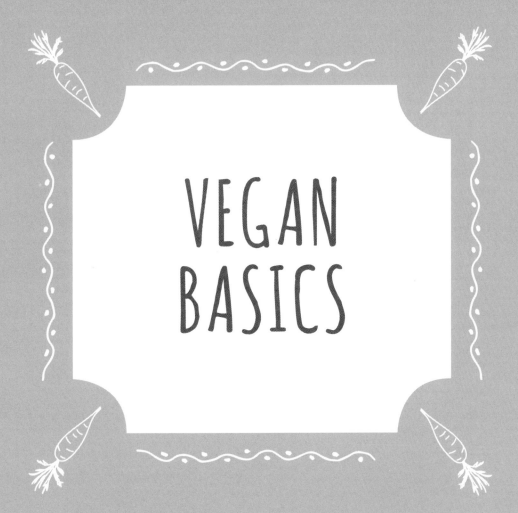

VEGAN BASICS

MYTH-BUSTING

Adopting a vegan diet is a personal choice and is often based on nutrition, animal welfare, or the environment. As with many alternative dietary choices, there are some common misconceptions. Here, the top myths that surround veganism are dispelled.

A VEGAN DIET IS EXPENSIVE!

IT DOESN'T HAVE TO BE... As with all diets, the cost greatly depends on how much you cook from scratch. The most efficient way to economize is to plan your weekly cooking and shop accordingly. Expensive convenience foods can be avoided. Instead, rely on fresh produce. You will actually be making a saving by not buying meat and fish, as they can be expensive. Instead, gradually build up a store cupboard of dried goods. This means you can always make a meal on a budget.

IT'S NOT HEALTHY!

YES, IT CAN BE... What constitutes healthy for anyone is a varied and broad diet, and many non-vegan diets may be very unhealthy if nutrition isn't considered. Vegans have the same nutritional needs as everyone else, so think about balance, eating a variety of colours, and ensuring you get enough of all the food groups. Protein is often a big worry as traditionally this comes from chicken, meat, fish, and dairy – but there are plenty of plant-based sources too.

VEGANS ARE ALWAYS TIRED

NO, THEY AREN'T... As long as you don't load up on convenience foods, you will have plenty of energy. You just need to ensure you are getting any nutrients typically found in animal products, such as calcium and iron, from other sources. Most nutrients can be easily replaced by plant-based sources and there are also lots of fortified products available.

VEGAN FOOD IS BORING

NO, IT ISN'T... People tend to think that a vegan diet consists of kale and salads. The reality is that a plant-based diet can be full of extremely tasty and varied food. It's best to focus on getting a range of fruits, vegetables, and other plant-based foods into your diet rather than think about what you'll be cutting out. The key is to experiment with flavour so your palate is sated; this way, you won't feel like something is missing. Season your food well to enhance the flavours.

THE FOOD IS DIFFICULT TO PREPARE!

IT CERTAINLY ISN'T... Vegan cooking can actually be easier than cooking with meat, fish, or dairy, as vegetables are very forgiving and adaptable. Cooking techniques are also largely the same, making the transition easy. Roasting, griddling, and barbecuing will draw out the best flavours from some vegetables, and grilling, poaching, or steaming can be used for fresher flavours. The only difficulty really lies in being adventurous, but this can be taken slowly. Start by adapting nostalgic comfort foods and gradually build up your recipe repertoire.

IT'S IMPOSSIBLE TO EAT OUT!

NOT ANYMORE... Eating out is no longer a problem, as many places now offer a vegan option and there are increasing numbers of purely vegan restaurants. Many world cuisines have dishes that are traditionally vegan or can be easily adapted. Chinese restaurants have lots of tofu and vegetable dishes to choose from, but be on the alert for hidden fish-based pastes and sauces – it is always wise to ask. Indian cuisine often has lentil or vegetable specialities, but watch out for ghee and yogurt used in the cooking. Many Thai dishes are vegan, but ask, as some dishes contain hidden scrambled eggs!

THE BALANCED VEGAN DIET

For new vegans, one major concern is ensuring you get the nutrients you need. Vegans have the same basic nutritional needs as everyone else, but they need to adjust the proportions of each food group. The key is balancing everything so you remain strong, energized, and in good health. This means making sense of what a healthy vegan meal is comprised of and building up a nourishing repertoire of dishes.

EVERYONE'S DAILY NEEDS

NUTRITION NEEDS VARY depending on your sex, size, age, and activity levels. As individuals, we all have varying requirements for energy and nutrients. This chart is a general guide to daily recommended amounts for a moderately active adult, whether following a vegan diet or not.

	MEN	WOMEN
ENERGY (KCAL)	2500	2000
PROTEIN (g)	55	50
CARBOHYDRATES (g)	300	260
SUGAR (g)	120	90
FAT (g)	95	70
SATURATES (g)	30	20
SALT (g)	6	6

30g fibre a day is recommended by health experts

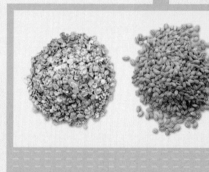

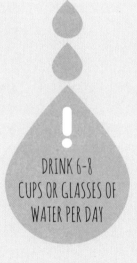

DRINK 6-8 CUPS OR GLASSES OF WATER PER DAY

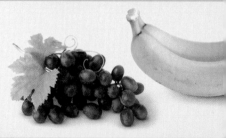

Aim to eat 3–4 servings of fruit daily.

1 serving = 1 piece or about 85g (3oz)

FRUIT

These include avocados, nuts, and dairy substitutes such as almond and soy. Don't overdo it.

1 serving = 30g (1oz) of nuts, ½ avocado

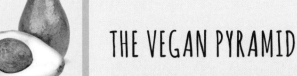

HIGH-FAT WHOLEFOODS

THE VEGAN PYRAMID

THIS MODIFIED, VEGAN VERSION of the food group pyramid is a great starting point for getting balance and variety into a plant-based diet. It is only a general guide, so don't worry if you can't get all of the food groups in every day – sometimes this may not be practical if you're busy or you have other foods to eat up in the fridge. As long as you practise eating a variety of different healthy foods it will all balance out over the week.

Broccoli, cabbage, spinach, and kale are good examples. Eat at least 2–3 servings daily.

1 serving = 85g (3oz) uncooked

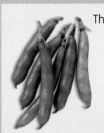

These protein-packed foods include beans, peas, and lentils. Eat 2–3 servings per day.

1 serving = palm of your hand, about 125g (4½oz)

LEAFY GREENS   ## LEGUMES

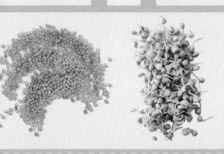

Brown rice, quinoa, buckwheat, barley, farro, wholegrain pasta, and sprouted grains are good choices. Always choose unrefined carbs, as these are high in fibre. Eat 5 or more servings per day.

1 serving = 30g (1oz) grains or 1 slice of wholemeal bread

WHOLEGRAINS

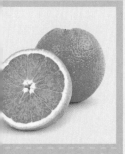

You can't eat too much veg! Eat as many different colours as possible each day.

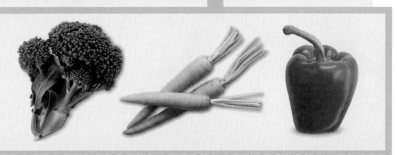

VEGETABLES

KEY MACRONUTRIENTS

Macronutrients are the nutrients needed in large amounts by the body to provide the bulk of your energy – they are the caloric building blocks of food. They are divided into fat, carbohydrates, and protein (see pp12–13 for the recommended daily amounts of each). Many vegans worry about protein, as this traditionally comes from meat, fish, and dairy, but there are plenty of great plant-based sources too.

FAT

A CERTAIN AMOUNT OF FAT is essential for the body to function, and it helps it absorb vitamins A, D, and E. Unhealthy saturated fats are mainly derived from animal products, so you're benefiting from cutting these out, but the healthier unsaturated fats play an important part in a healthy vegan diet. Seeds and nuts are a great source of unsaturated fats, such as the healthy fatty acid omega-3. The body doesn't need a huge amount of fat, so watch your intake of fatty foods – even the healthy ones!

GOOD PLANT-BASED SOURCES OF UNSATURATED FATS
Healthy fats are found in foods such as avocados, almonds, walnuts, cashew nuts, Brazil nuts, pumpkin seeds, chia seeds, olive oil, winter squash, leafy greens, and members of the cabbage family.

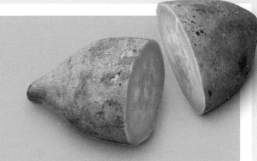

CARBOHYDRATES

CARBOHYDRATES ARE the main energy source for our body, so it is necessary to include them to avoid fatigue and anxiety. They are fairly easy to come by in a vegan diet; the trick is to stick to eating the healthiest sources. You don't have to load up on bread and potatoes – many fruits, vegetables, and wholegrains are carbs too.

GOOD PLANT-BASED SOURCES OF CARBS
Fruits and vegetables such as bananas, broccoli, apples, sweet potatoes, leafy greens, carrots, figs, and squash. Wholegrains such as wild rice, wholemeal rice, and oats.

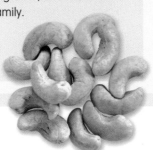

PROTEIN

PROTEIN BUILDS MUSCLE, cells, and tissue and produces hormones and antibodies. It is made up of 20 amino acids, of which nine are essential, as we can't make these ourselves. As a vegan, you need to make sure to eat a variety of different protein sources to get all the amino acids your body needs. Below are some of the best plant-based sources.

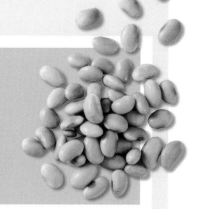

GRAINS

- BUCKWHEAT 175g (6oz) provides 22.5g of protein.
- COOKED WILD RICE 185g (6½oz) provides 6.5g of protein.
- QUINOA 185g (6½oz) provides 8g of protein.

LEGUMES

- COOKED BLACK BEANS A 30g (1oz) serving will provide 7.5g of protein and is packed with B6. Good for slow-releasing energy.
- COOKED ORGANIC EDAMAME BEANS A 15g (½oz) serving provides high-quality protein with all the essential amino acids. Eating 200g (7oz) will provide you with about 22g of protein, nearly half the daily recommended amount.
- LENTILS A 100g (3½oz) serving will provide 9g of protein. As lentils are high in fibre and low in calories, they are good for slow-releasing energy.
- ORGANIC TEMPEH A 75g (2½oz) serving will provide 16g of protein.
- ORGANIC TOFU A 75g (2½oz) serving will provide 8-15g of protein. This is a similar protein content to chicken. It will keep you full for hours. Spreadable varieties taste good on oatcakes.
- PEANUT BUTTER 2 tbsp will provide 7g of protein.
- PEANUTS A 60g (2oz) serving will provide 7g of protein. Great for snacking on.

SEEDS

- CHIA SEEDS 2 tbsp provides 4g of protein.
- HEMP SEEDS 3 tbsp provides 10g of protein.

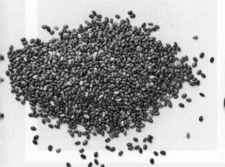
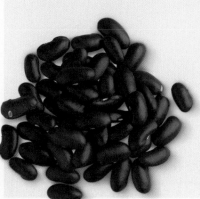
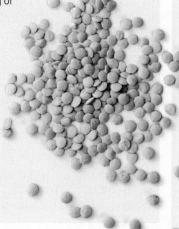

VITAL VITAMINS

A group of micronutrients found in different types of food, vitamins are essential for our body's growth, vitality, and for general wellbeing. Most of these can be gained from a balanced vegan diet, although you may need supplement B12 and D. The Bs and vitamin C need to be consumed each day as the body cannot store them. The wheel highlights the function of each vitamin and the best sources for vegans.

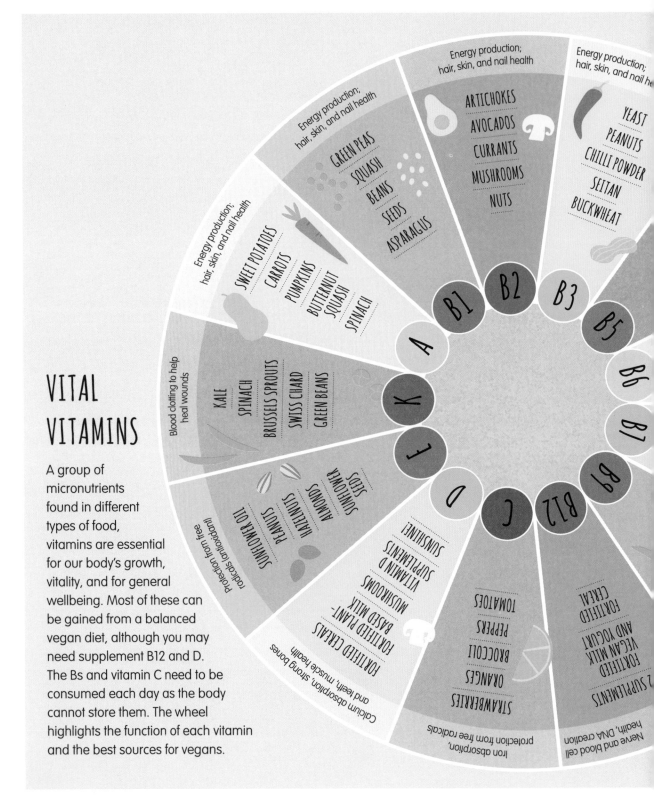

Energy production; hair, skin, and nail health

GREEN PEAS
SQUASH
BEANS
SEEDS
ASPARAGUS

Energy production; hair, skin, and nail health

ARTICHOKES
AVOCADOS
CURRANTS
MUSHROOMS
NUTS

Energy production; hair, skin, and nail health

YEAST
PEANUTS
CHILLI POWDER
SEITAN
BUCKWHEAT

Energy production; hair, skin, and nail health

SWEET POTATOES
CARROTS
PUMPKINS
BUTTERNUT SQUASH
SPINACH

Blood clotting to help heal wounds

KALE
SPINACH
BRUSSELS SPROUTS
SWISS CHARD
GREEN BEANS

Protection from free radicals (antioxidant)

SUNFLOWER OIL
PEANUTS
HAZELNUTS
ALMONDS
SUNFLOWER SEEDS

Calcium absorption, strong bones and teeth, muscle health

FORTIFIED CEREALS
FORTIFIED PLANT-BASED MILK
MUSHROOMS
VITAMIN D SUPPLEMENTS
SUNSHINE!

Iron absorption, protection from free radicals

STRAWBERRIES
ORANGES
BROCCOLI
PEPPERS
TOMATOES

Nerve and blood cell health, DNA creation

B12 SUPPLEMENTS
FORTIFIED VEGAN MILK AND YOGURT
FORTIFIED CEREAL

A B1 B2 B3 B5 B6 B7 B9 B12 C D E K

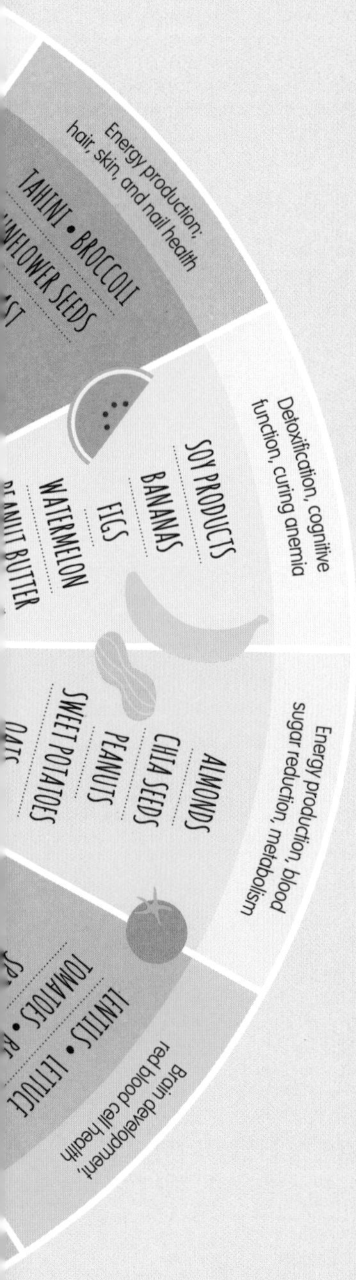

VITAMINS AND MINERALS

Vitamins and minerals are the two types of micronutrients. They are needed in smaller amounts than macronutrients but are equally as important to our wellbeing. They help to regulate metabolism, the heart, and bone density.

(wheel, left margin — rotated text)

Energy production; hair, skin, and nail health

TAHINI • BROCCOLI

SUNFLOWER SEEDS

YEAST

Detoxification, cognitive function, curing anemia

SOY PRODUCTS

BANANAS

FIGS

WATERMELON

PEANUT BUTTER

Energy production, blood sugar reduction, metabolism

ALMONDS

CHIA SEEDS

PEANUTS

SWEET POTATOES

OATS

Brain development, red blood cell health

TOMATOES

LENTILS • LETTUCE

MUST-HAVE MINERALS

Minerals help with bone and tooth formation, blood coagulation, and muscle contraction. They are divided into macro minerals and trace minerals. Your body needs macro minerals in much larger amounts than trace minerals. As long as you eat a varied, balanced plant-based diet, you'll get plenty of most minerals. However, there are a few exceptions you should watch out for.

MACRO MINERALS

calcium, chlorine, magnesium, phosphorus, potassium, sodium, and sulphur.

CALCIUM A big worry for some when not consuming dairy is "where will my calcium come from?" Calcium can be found in dark leafy greens, fortified plant milk, soy products, nuts, and seeds, as well as some fruit such as blackberries, blackcurrants, oranges, and figs.

TRACE MINERALS

chromium, cobalt, copper, fluorine, iodine, iron, manganese, molybdenum, selenium, and zinc.

IRON As red meat is the most common source of iron, vegans need to look elsewhere for good plant-based sources. There are plenty of iron-rich vegan options such as lentils, chickpeas, beans, tofu, cashew nuts, spinach, ground linseed, kale, raisins, fortified breakfast cereal, and quinoa.

IODINE Our body needs iodine to make thyroid hormones. Often sourced from dairy, vegan milk options don't contain adequate levels of it so you need to include iodine-rich foods in your diet. Cranberries or cranberry juice, strawberries, haricot and butter beans, potatoes baked in skins, and seaweed are all good sources.

VEGAN SUBSTITUTES

It can be overwhelming at first to embark on a plant-based diet, but with all the substitutes that are available, the transition can be made much simpler. Easy vegan swaps can now be found for most familiar foods in supermarkets, making the weekly shop less intimidating and the cooking far easier.

MILK

For many new vegans, finding a good milk alternative is the most important swap. The decision is often down to taste preferences, but it is also worth comparing the nutritional benefits of plant-based milks.

ALMOND MILK	Almond milk is a popular choice for flavour. It is usually fortified with calcium, but is not a great source of protein or fibre. Best for overall cooking – but the flavour can overpower in baking.
COCONUT MILK	Coconut milk is lower in calories than other plant-based milks, but it is not naturally nutritionally packed unless it is fortified. It contains virtually no protein.
OAT MILK	Oat milk is the best choice for fibre, but low in protein and high in carbohydrates and calories. It has a decent amount of calcium and iron and naturally contains B vitamins that soya and almond milk don't. It is a good option for those with soya or nut allergies and good for baking.
SOYA MILK	Soya milk is the most protein-rich option, and nutritionally the most similar to cow's milk. However, it doesn't contain huge amounts of calcium, iodine, or B vitamins unless added. Drink sparingly if you already eat a lot of other soy products. Soya milk makes the best latte!

BUTTER

Plant-based margarine can be substituted weight for weight in recipes. Olive-oil-based versions are good for shallow frying and spreading and are lower in calories than other margarines. Soya spread is also good for general cooking, and sunflower spread works well for baking.

YOGURT

Vegan soya yogurt is a great dairy yogurt alternative; it also tends to react in a similar way when cooking. Coconut yogurt supplies several key vitamins and minerals and can have live and active cultures just like milk-based yogurts.

CHEESE

Nutritional yeast is a good substitute, especially for baking, as it offers a savoury cheese flavour and it is rich in B vitamins. Vegan versions of most cheeses are also now widely available. It's probably best to try out a few different types and brands, as it's all down to personal taste.

EGGS

Eggs are invaluable for baking, but the starchy water from canned chickpeas and beans (aquafaba) is full of protein and can be used as the perfect egg replacement. It has emulsifying, binding, foaming, and thickening properties and performs as egg whites do when whipped – making it the ideal ingredient to make meringues. It is best to use the water straight from the can of chickpeas. A regular 400ml (14fl oz) can has about 12 tbsp of aquafaba. As a rule of thumb, 3 tbsp of aquafaba = 1 whole egg and 2 tbsp = 1 egg white.

HONEY

Replacing honey in a recipe is fairly simple. You can generally swap the honey quantity for the same amount of agave, which is a concentrated sweetener with a similar texture to honey. Maple syrup also makes a good swap, as it has a similar texture and is good for drizzling. Maple syrup has a slightly stronger flavour than agave and the really good stuff can be quite expensive, but a little goes a long way.

MEAT

Seitan, tempeh, and tofu are the major meat alternatives, all of which can be bought in their natural form or marinated with added flavours. Many recipes will also replace meat with filling grains, pulses, and nuts.

SEITAN	Seitan is a non-soy product. Its texture and its ability to absorb flavours make it a good meat substitute. It is made by washing wheat flour dough with water until all the starch has been removed. This leaves the dense, elastic gluten which can be baked, sautéed, steamed, or stewed. It is high in protein and low in calories, but can't be eaten by anyone with wheat allergies or following a gluten-free diet.
TEMPEH	Tempeh is made by fermenting soya beans, a process that ups the protein content to rival meat. Tempeh is even healthier than tofu as the fermentation helps to break down anti-nutrients found in soya beans, making its proteins more digestible. It is also high in vitamins B5, B6, B3, and B2. Tempeh is good for grilling, frying, and roasting and makes a great bacon substitute.
TOFU	Tofu is also called bean curd. It is made by curdling and pressing soya milk (made from soya beans) into the blocks of tofu that you can buy. It is low in fat and calories and high in protein and amino acids. Firm tofu is good for using in stir-fries and soups, as it keeps its structure.

TIPS FOR MAKING THE SWITCH

The switch to a plant-based diet can be smooth running, but to make sure it works for you, it needs to fit into your lifestyle. You may need more time to prep main meals and snacks, investigate nutrition, and change your shopping habits. It doesn't have to be all or nothing – you can make changes at your own pace. Whatever the transition, eating a plant-based diet will eventually become a natural part of your life.

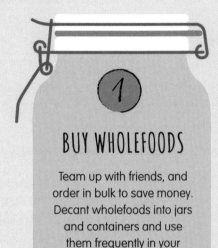

1
BUY WHOLEFOODS
Team up with friends, and order in bulk to save money. Decant wholefoods into jars and containers and use them frequently in your favourite recipes.

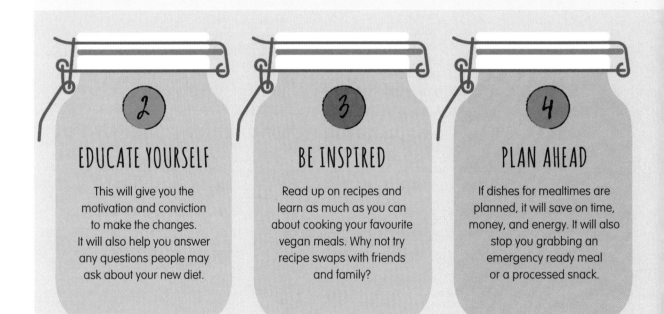

2
EDUCATE YOURSELF
This will give you the motivation and conviction to make the changes. It will also help you answer any questions people may ask about your new diet.

3
BE INSPIRED
Read up on recipes and learn as much as you can about cooking your favourite vegan meals. Why not try recipe swaps with friends and family?

4
PLAN AHEAD
If dishes for mealtimes are planned, it will save on time, money, and energy. It will also stop you grabbing an emergency ready meal or a processed snack.

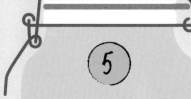

5 BATCH COOK

Cook one for now and one for the freezer. This will free up time when the family is busy or when you're too tired to start cooking a big meal.

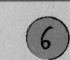

6 MAKE FAMILY FAVOURITES

Learn to make healthy vegan versions of favourite takeaways or junk food, such as burgers, Chinese food, or pies.

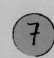

7 TAKE A SUPPLEMENT

It will offer reassurance that you are getting the nutrients you need.

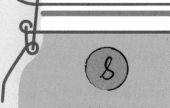

8 DRINK FLUIDS

Healthy fluids such as water and herbal teas are great for keeping you hydrated and alleviating hunger pangs – we are often thirsty when we think we are hungry!

9 EXPERIMENT

Get creative in the kitchen as much as you can, trying new flavour combinations and cooking methods. This keeps a vegan diet exciting. Don't be afraid of failures!

10 FILL THE FRIDGE

Make sure your fridge is packed with healthy vegan snacks and remove any over-processed foods to avoid temptation.

THE YOUNG VEGAN

A vegan diet can be suitable for all ages, but as with any restrictive diet, it is wise to consult a dietician or nutritionist before making the transition so no compromises are made and daily nutritional targets are met. It is ideal for children to learn about diet as early on as possible so they can continue to make informed healthy choices as they get older.

GROWING CHILDREN

CHILDREN GROW RAPIDLY from toddler to 12, so they need a diet that provides adequate amounts of protein to calorie ratio for energy and development. The best thing you can do for your vegan children is to introduce them to as many flavours and textures as early on as you can, which will develop the palate so they become more adventurous. Children eating a healthy plant-based diet will be far more nourished than children growing up on junk food, but in order to provide this, you need to be mindful of any particularly important nutrients or specific adjustments for kids.

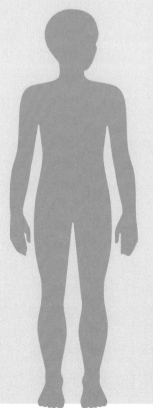

VITAMIN D

Children need a lot of vitamin D, the sunshine vitamin, for healthy bone growth. Make sure they get plenty from fortified cereals.

IRON

Make sure your child gets enough iron from a plant-based diet. Iron gives red blood cells the "strength" to carry oxygen in the body, which is vital for children's growth.

FIBRE
Vegan diets can be too high in fibre for young children, so they tend to feel full up before they've eaten enough nutrients. Try giving them some white bread, pasta, and rice instead of brown.

CALCIUM
Calcium is vital for growing bones and teeth. This typically comes from dairy products, but many plant-based alternatives and cereals are fortified with calcium.

FUEL FOR TEENAGERS

TEENS NEED TO EAT at least three nutritious meals a day, a couple of healthy snacks, and plenty of water. Teenage boys need 2,500 calories a day and girls 2,000. Skipping meals only leads to bad eating habits and unhealthy snacking. Food also play a vital role in concentration, so teens need to eat regularly to keep blood sugars from dropping and the brain from becoming foggy. They should fill up on nutrient-dense wholefoods that will help the body thrive physically and mentally. There are some nutrients that you need more of as you go into your teenage years.

5 QUICK ENERGY BOOSTS FOR KIDS

- TROPICAL FRUIT SMOOTHIE BOWL (pp40-41)
- PEANUT BUTTER & BANANA BALLS (pp54-55)
- LEMONY SPINACH HUMMUS (pp64-65)
- CHICKPEA BITES (p66)
- MUNG BEAN GUACAMOLE (pp70-71)

IRON

The need for iron increases in teenagers as their muscle mass increases and blood volume expands. It is recommended that teenage boys get on average 11 milligrams of iron a day and girls get 15 milligrams a day. Not getting enough iron can lead to anemia, which will result in fatigue, headaches and light headedness, and an inability to concentrate.

PROTEIN

Protein requirements increase for teens because of metabolic changes, growth spurts, and high activity. Their needs should be met if they eat a varied diet with plenty of legumes, seeds, and wholegrains.

CALCIUM

Calcium is especially important for teens because it's a period of major growth spurts. Make sure teens are consuming enough calcium to prevent the future risk of osteoporosis – consuming adequate calcium during the teenage years reduces the risk of brittle bones later in life.

VITAMIN C

It is a good idea for teens to be particularly careful to eat foods rich in vitamin C as part of their meals, as this vitamin helps the body absorb more iron.

SHOPPING FOR VEGAN FOODS

Whether you or your family are transitioning into eating a wholly plant-based diet or you are going to do it a few steps at a time, your shopping habits will begin to change. If you are strapped for time, it makes sense to research ahead of supermarket trips so time isn't wasted.

LABEL READING

IT'S EASY TO shop for fresh fruits and vegetables, but it can get tricky with non-perishables. Many products now clearly state if they are vegan, but it is wise to know the non-vegan sneaky ingredients that might catch you out.

- **ALBUMEN** comes from eggs.

- **ASPIC** comes from clarified meat or fish or from gelatin.

- **CASEIN** is milk protein.

- **COD LIVER OIL** comes from a cod's liver.

- **COLLAGEN** comes from the skin, bones, or connective tissue of animals.

- **DAIRY AND EGGS** are allergens, so these will be clearly stated on the label and any by-products will be highlighted.

- **ELASTIN** is similar to collagen, but comes from the neck ligaments of cows.

- **E NUMBERS** are food additives and may contain things like cochineal (a dye made from beetles).

- **GELATIN** is derived from the boiled bones, skin, and ligaments of cows or pigs.

- **HONEY** is produced by bees.

- **ISINGLASS** comes from the bladder of fish (may be used in refining wine and beer).

- **KERATIN** comes from the skin, bones, or connective tissue of animals.

- **LACTOSE** is a milk sugar.

- **LARD/TALLOW** is animal fat.

- **PEPSIN** comes from a pig's stomach.

- **PROPOLIS** is used by bees to make their hives.

- **ROYAL JELLY** is a secretion from the honey bee.

- **SHELLAC** comes from the body of a female insect.

- **VITAMIN D3** is sometimes derived from fish liver or sheep's wool (lanolin). It can be vegan if made from lichen. Always check the label!

- **WHEY** is a milk by-product.

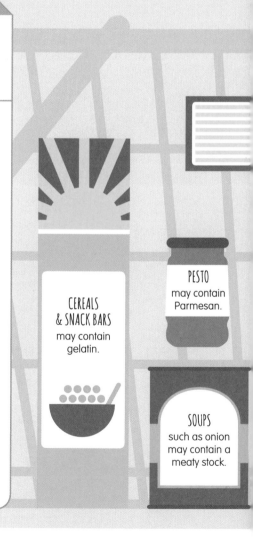

CEREALS & SNACK BARS may contain gelatin.

PESTO may contain Parmesan.

SOUPS such as onion may contain a meaty stock.

PRODUCTS TO WATCH OUT FOR

SOME FOODS appear vegan at first glance but actually contain hidden animal products. You can find vegan versions of many of these, but you can't assume! Below are a few key products to watch out for.

TIP

LOOK OUT FOR TRUSTED VEGAN REGISTERED TRADEMARKS ON PRODUCTS TO GIVE YOU REASSURANCE.

MARSHMALLOWS & JELLY
products will usually contain gelatin.

RED & GREEN THAI CURRY PASTE
may contain fish sauce or dried shrimp.

BREADS
may contain milk powder or whey.

FRESH PASTA
contains egg – most dried doesn't, but best to check.

SALAD DRESSING
may contain emulsifiers and egg yolk. Caesar dressing contains anchovies.

BREAD & DOUGH
products may contain L-Cysteine, an added amino acid that comes from duck feathers or hog hair.

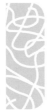

NOODLES
will often contain egg. Rice noodles, as well as some soba noodles, are a good choice.

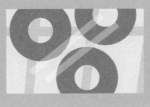

MARGARINE
is not always vegan. It may contain whey, gelatin, or milk proteins.

CRISPS
may contain milk powder.

WINE & BEER
may have been refined using isinglass – check the label.

ORANGE JUICE
may have added lanolin-based vitamin D3.

WORCESTERSHIRE SAUCE
contains anchovies.

STOCKING YOUR VEGAN KITCHEN

Having a well-stocked vegan store cupboard and freezer really saves time
and makes food prep easier, as so many plant-based items are non-perishable.
Buy these ingredients regularly so you can whip up a meal at a moment's
notice with the addition of some fresh produce.

NUTS AND SEEDS To keep these fresh, buy nuts and seeds in small quantities. Once open, keep in an airtight glass jar and away from sunlight. Whole nuts will keep much longer than shelled and ground. Pecans, peanuts, and walnuts will spoil the quickest, so keep in the fridge. Cashews and whole almonds will last the longest. Store seeds in jars in the fridge for ultimate freshness.

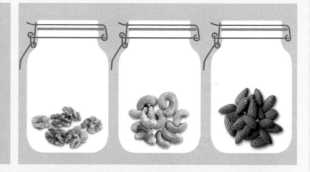

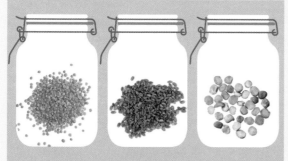

DRIED BEANS, PULSES, AND LENTILS With their long shelf life, these are invaluable for the vegan pantry. Once opened, keep in jars away from sunlight. Stock a mix of red, white, and black beans. Dried beans need soaking for 6-8 hours, so plan meals ahead. Lentils don't require soaking, making them the perfect convenience food. Also stock up on canned beans and cooked lentil pouches for ease.

GRAINS Wholegrains are essential for the vegan diet; bulgur wheat, quinoa, farro, and pearl barley are all great examples. Store in glass jars away from sunlight.

RICE Store a selection of brown, white basmati, red, wild, and arborio rice. A great vegan food to stock up on; when kept in a sealed container, rice will keep for years.

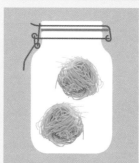

NOODLES AND PASTA You can store dried, egg-free versions of both noodles and pasta in your cupboard for 1-2 years. Choose wholemeal pasta for higher fibre.

MAXIMIZING YOUR FREEZER

A GREAT WAY to save time and money is to batch cook meals for the freezer. This will make it much easier to maintain a new diet. Meals such as chillies, curries, and soups even get tastier as the flavours are left to mingle. Freezing key ingredients for vegan cooking is also a great time-saving trick. Below are the best foods to freeze.

WHOLEMEAL BREADCRUMBS	LAST 3 MONTHS	Lots of vegan recipes need breadcrumbs for thickening or binding. Save all leftover bread and whizz in a food processor in one batch. Seal in a container and freeze. These can be used from frozen.
CHICKPEAS AND BEANS	LAST 1 YEAR	Having dried chickpeas or beans soaked, cooked, and frozen in portion sizes is invaluable for the busy cook. You can then stir them straight into dishes or run under warm water if wanting to blend.
AVOCADOS	LAST 1 YEAR	It's good to stock avocados, especially if they are in danger of not being eaten in time. Peel, stone, and quarter, then open freeze on trays before putting into freezer bags. Remove and thaw before use.
NUTS AND FLOUR	LAST 1 MONTH	Freezing will keep these fresher for longer, so a good solution if you buy in bulk. Portion into plastic freezer bags. Use them straight from the freezer. For ground nuts, blitz in a food processor first, then freeze.
HERBS AND SPICES	LAST 1 YEAR	Buy difficult-to-find herbs and spices when you see them. These are great for adding exciting flavours to plant-based dishes. Freeze in small sealable bags and use straight from the freezer.
AQUAFABA	LASTS 1 MONTH	Thaw before use. Use to whip up meringues or use for cakes and bakes as an egg replacement. Freeze in your required portion sizes or in ice cube trays, then transfer to a sealable freezer bag.

DAY 2

BREAKFAST
Berry & chia smoothie bowl
(pp38-39)

LUNCH
Quesadillas with pinto beans & sweet potato
(pp132-33)

DINNER
Vegetable stir-fry (pp168-69)

SNACKS
Apple slices dipped into peanut butter,
Tropical immune boosters
(pp62-63)

DAY 1

BREAKFAST
Superseed granola (pp34-35)

LUNCH
Sweet potato, teff, & peanut soup (pp100-01)

DINNER
Three bean paella (pp156-57)

SNACKS
Tropical immune boosters (pp62-63),
Avocado & banana recovery
bites (pp56-57)

DAY 3

BREAKFAST
Avocado, nori, & nut cream toasts
(pp36-37)

LUNCH
Creamy green soup
(pp88-89)

DINNER
Rainbow lentil meatballs (pp146-47)

SNACKS
Mung bean guacamole (pp70-71),
Raw energy bars (pp58-59)

DAY 4

BREAKFAST
Wholewheat banana pecan
pancakes (p51)

LUNCH
Vermicelli rice noodles (pp142-43)

DINNER
Sweet potato & spinach curry (pp162-63)

SNACKS
Carrot sticks and radish with plant-based
yogurt, Raw energy bars (pp58-59)

7 DAY MEAL PLAN

THIS IS A GREAT STARTING point
for new vegans. These simple
but tasty recipes will provide
variation and all the nutrients
you need over a week.

MEAL PLANNING

Planning your meals is a great way to make eating or cooking a plant-based diet much easier. A meal plan for the week is simple; you can stick to what you feel comfortable with at first and then get more creative as you become more confident. Having your ingredients in the fridge and a recipe at the ready will also ensure you don't make bad food decisions when you are hungry. Meal planning ahead can also be an economical way of eating.

DAY 5

BREAKFAST
Oat & almond milk porridge (pp42-43)

LUNCH
Brown rice risotto with peppers and artichokes (pp160-61)

DINNER
Udon noodles with sweet and sour tofu (p149)

SNACKS
Handful of almonds and dried apricots, Chickpea bites (p66)

DAY 6

BREAKFAST
Yellow lentil waffles (pp32-33)

LUNCH
Seitan gyros (pp126-27)

DINNER
Root vegetable stew (pp108-09)

SNACKS
Lemony spinach hummus (pp64-65), Chickpea bites (p66)

DAY 7

BREAKFAST
Ancient grains porridge with pear (pp48-49)

LUNCH
Brown rice sushi bowl (pp174-75)

DINNER
Turkish stuffed aubergine (pp204-05)

SNACKS
Garlicky onion crackers (pp68-69) with Cashew ricotta (p66) Peanut butter & banana balls (pp54-55)

BREAKFAST & BRUNCH

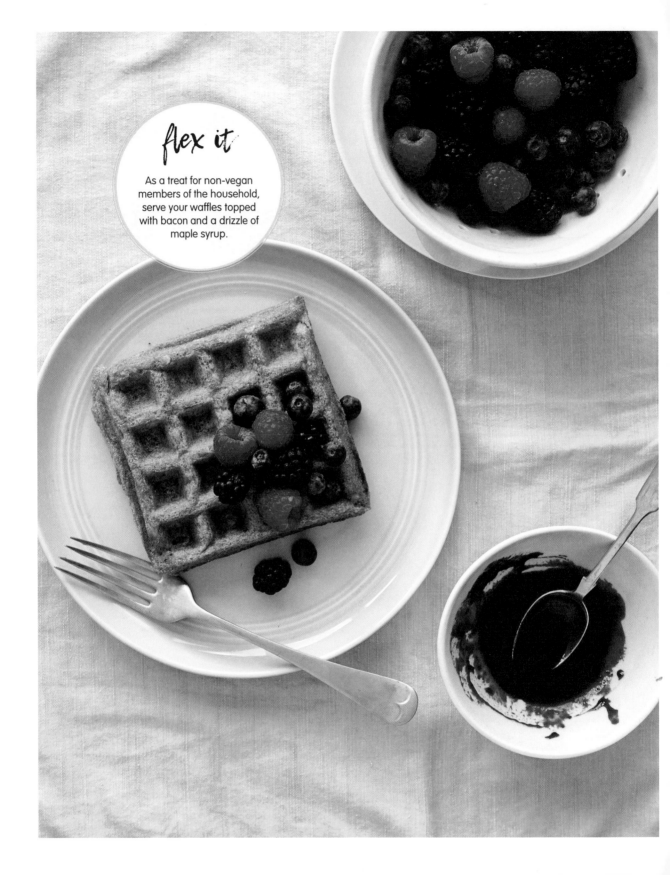

flex it

As a treat for non-vegan members of the household, serve your waffles topped with bacon and a drizzle of maple syrup.

YELLOW LENTIL WAFFLES
with five-spice berry sauce

SERVES 4
PREP 15 MINS
COOK 15 MINS

175g (6oz) **raspberries**
175g (6oz) **blackberries**
175g (6oz) **blueberries**
¼ tsp **five-spice powder**
1 **cinnamon stick**
300ml (10fl oz) **unsweetened almond milk**
60ml (2fl oz) **rapeseed oil**
2 tsp **vanilla extract**
3 tbsp **agave nectar**
225g (8oz) **wholemeal flour**
1½ tsp **baking powder**
115g (4oz) cooked **yellow lentils**

1 In a small saucepan, combine the raspberries, blackberries, blueberries, five-spice powder, and cinnamon stick. Cover and cook over a low heat for 15 minutes, stirring regularly, until the berries break down into a thickened sauce. Add 2–3 tablespoons of water as needed.

2 Meanwhile, in a small bowl whisk together the almond milk, oil, vanilla, and agave.

3 Preheat a waffle maker. In a large mixing bowl, combine the flour and baking powder. Incorporate the almond milk mixture into the flour mixture. Gently fold in the lentils.

4 When the waffle iron is hot, spray it with cooking spray. Add 120ml (4fl oz) batter to each section and cook, according to the manufacturer's instructions, to make 4 waffles in total.

5 Remove the cinnamon stick from the sauce. Serve the waffles and sauce immediately.

the good stuff

The benefits of including lentils in your diet are numerous – they are high in protein but low in calories, so make a great healthy, filling breakfast food. They also contain high levels of soluble fibre to help lower cholesterol and reduce the risk of heart disease.

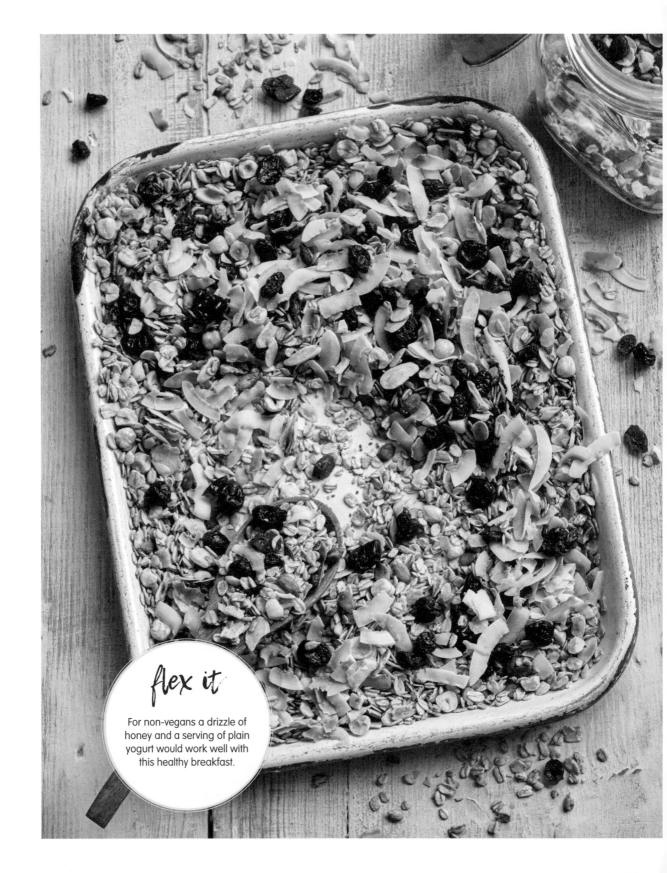

flex it

For non-vegans a drizzle of honey and a serving of plain yogurt would work well with this healthy breakfast.

SUPERSEED GRANOLA
with nuts, dried fruit, & chia seeds

SERVES 12
PREP 15 MINS
COOK 30–35 MINS

30g (1oz) **coconut oil**
75ml (2½fl oz) **maple syrup**
¼ tsp **fine salt**
1 tsp **ground cinnamon**
300g (10oz) **rolled oats**
30g (1oz) **pumpkin seeds**
30g (1oz) **sunflower seeds**
75g (2½oz) **flaked almonds**
75g (2½oz) **hazelnuts**,
  roughly chopped
115g (4oz) **dried fruit**, such
  as **cranberries, cherries, raisins,**
  pitted dates, roughly chopped
30g (1oz) **toasted coconut chips**
1 tbsp **chia seeds**
1 tbsp **golden flax seeds**

1 Preheat the oven to 160°C (325°F/Gas 3). If the coconut oil is solid, melt it in a small saucepan. Once melted, remove it from the heat and whisk in the maple syrup, salt, and cinnamon.

2 Mix the oats, pumpkin seeds, sunflower seeds, and nuts together in a large bowl. Pour the maple syrup liquid over the dried mixture, and toss it very well to combine.

3 Spread the granola mixture over 2 large baking trays. Place in the centre of the oven and bake for 30–40 minutes, turning every 10 minutes. Ensure that the granola is spread out, so that it browns evenly. The granola is ready when it is golden-brown and crunchy.

4 Allow the granola to cool, then mix in the dried fruit, toasted coconut chips, chia seeds, and flaxseeds. Serve with dairy-free yogurt or a dairy-free milk, and fresh fruit. You can store the granola in an airtight container for up to 2 weeks.

the good stuff

Nourishing oats provide slow-releasing energy and help reduce levels of cholesterol in the blood. Nuts and seeds provide healthy unsaturated fats and essential B vitamins.

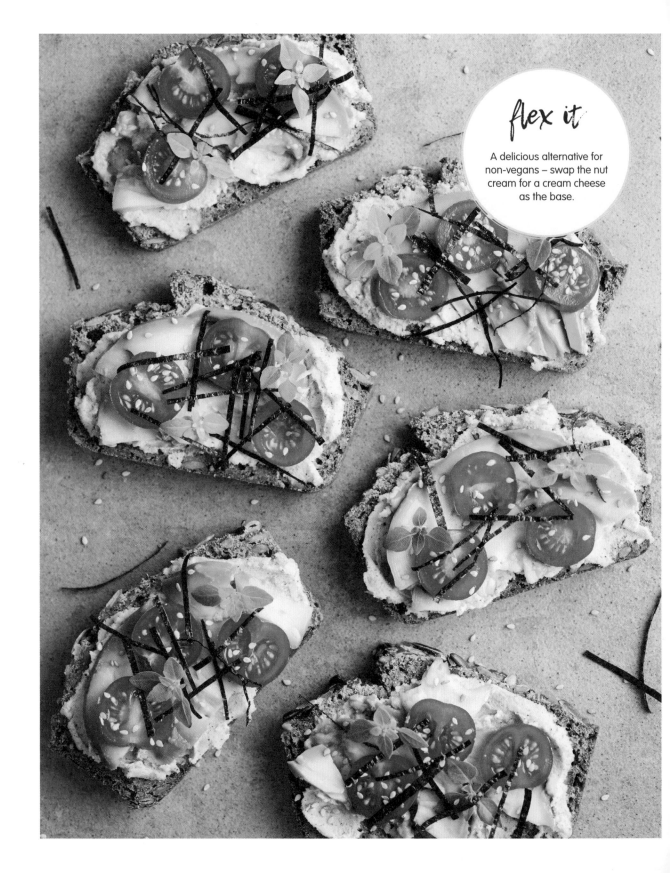

flex it

A delicious alternative for non-vegans – swap the nut cream for a cream cheese as the base.

AVOCADO, NORI, & NUT CREAM TOASTS
with sesame seeds & basil

SERVES 4
PREP 15 MINS

8 slices **quinoa superseed loaf**
1½ **avocados**, sliced
9 **cherry tomatoes**, sliced
3 tbsp **nori seaweed**, shredded
1 tbsp **sesame seeds**
a few sprigs of **basil**

NUT CREAM
115g (4oz) **Brazil nuts**
2 tbsp **lemon juice**
1 tbsp **olive oil**
salt and freshly ground
   black pepper

1 To make the nut cream, put the ingredients in a blender or processor, and whizz until combined. You may need to stop the machine occasionally to push the mixture down with a spatula. Gradually add 2 tablespoons of hot water to achieve a thick, creamy consistency. Season with salt and pepper.

2 Toast the bread and spread with nut cream. Top with the avocado, tomatoes, nori, seeds, and basil.

VARIATION

Top the nut cream with finely sliced radish, sliced cornichons, and sliced apple. Garnish with finely chopped dill.

the good stuff

Nori is packed with vitamin C and micronutrients such as iodine, which is essential as the body can't make it by itself – it is needed for the production of the thyroid hormone.

BERRY & CHIA SMOOTHIE BOWL
with mango & mulberries

SERVES 2
PREP 10 MINS

100g (3½oz) **frozen raspberries**
100g (3½oz) **frozen blueberries**
200ml (7fl oz) **nut milk**, such as almond
100g (3½oz) ripe **banana**
50g (1¾oz) **avocado**, sliced
2 tbsp **chia seeds**
2 tbsp **acai berry powder** (optional)

TOPPING
½ small **mango**, peeled and sliced
1 tbsp **flaked almonds**
20g (¾oz) **raspberries**
1 tbsp **pumpkin seeds**
1 tbsp **dried mulberries**

1 Put the smoothie ingredients in a high-speed blender or food processor and whizz until smooth. Transfer to 2 bowls.

2 Lay the mango slices in a starburst pattern over half the surface, then arrange the almonds, raspberries, pumpkin seeds, and mulberries in stripes on the other half.

VARIATION

Try adding 125g (4½oz) of raw beetroot (skin on) to the blender along with some chopped fresh ginger; if your smoothie is too thick, dilute it by adding more nut milk or add a little cold water.

the good stuff

A real power bowl for breakfast – the high potassium in bananas can protect you from workout muscle cramps, so this bowl is a good choice before morning exercise!

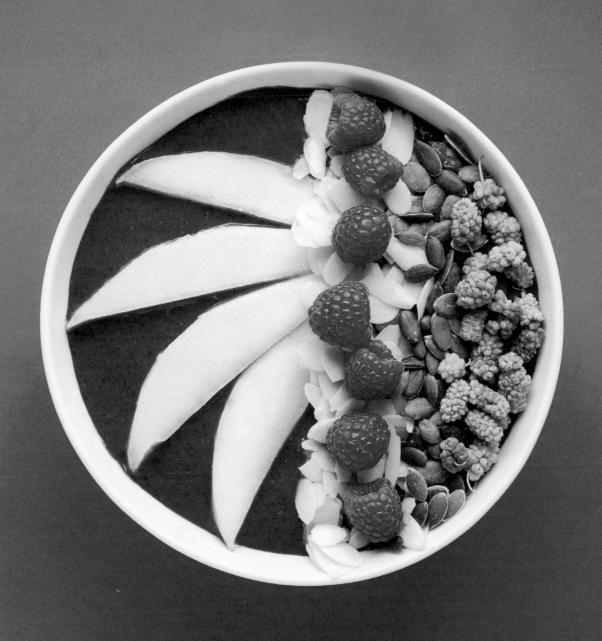

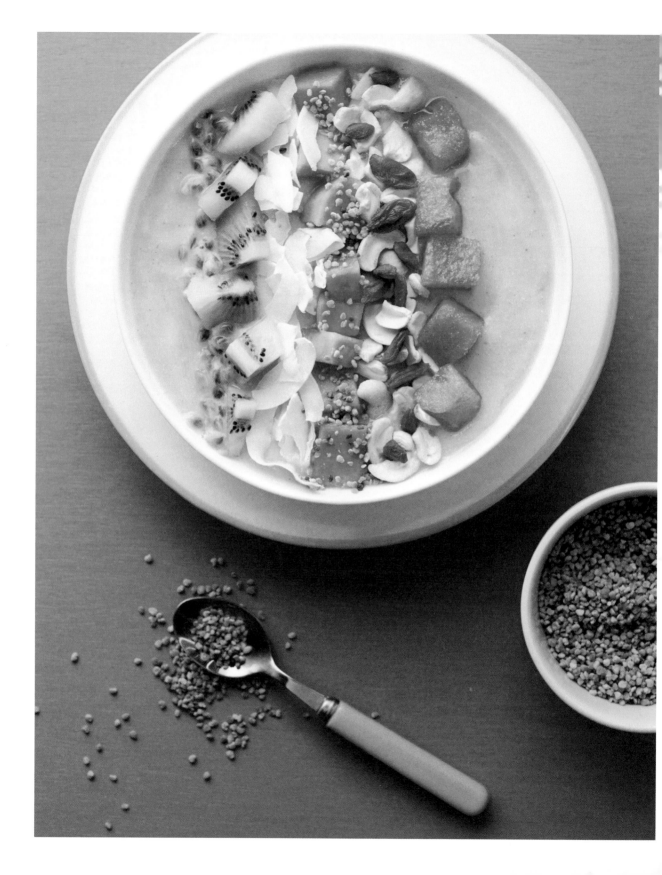

TROPICAL FRUIT SMOOTHIE BOWL
with coconut flakes & cashew nuts

SERVES 2
PREP 10 MINS

150g (5½oz) **frozen mango**
75g (2½oz) **frozen pineapple**
75g (2½oz) **papaya**
200ml (7fl oz) freshly squeezed
   orange juice (or shop bought)
2 tbsp **hemp seeds**
¼ tsp **ground turmeric**
1 tbsp **lucuma powder** (optional)

TOPPING
seeds of ½ **passion fruit**
½ **kiwi**, sliced
1 tbsp **coconut flakes**
1 small slice **papaya**, cut
   into chunks
1 tbsp **cashew nuts**
1 tsp **goji berries**
1 small slice **watermelon**, cut
   into chunks

1 Put the smoothie ingredients in a high-speed blender or food processor and whizz until smooth.

2 Pour into 2 bowls and arrange the toppings on the surface in stripes.

VARIATION

Try some other flavours that go with tropical fruits – add a handful of fresh mint and basil leaves to the blender along with a squeeze of lime.

the good stuff

This is great food to start the day. Mango, pineapple, and papaya are loaded with vitamin C, which will boost your immune system. Turmeric has powerful anti-inflammatory properties.

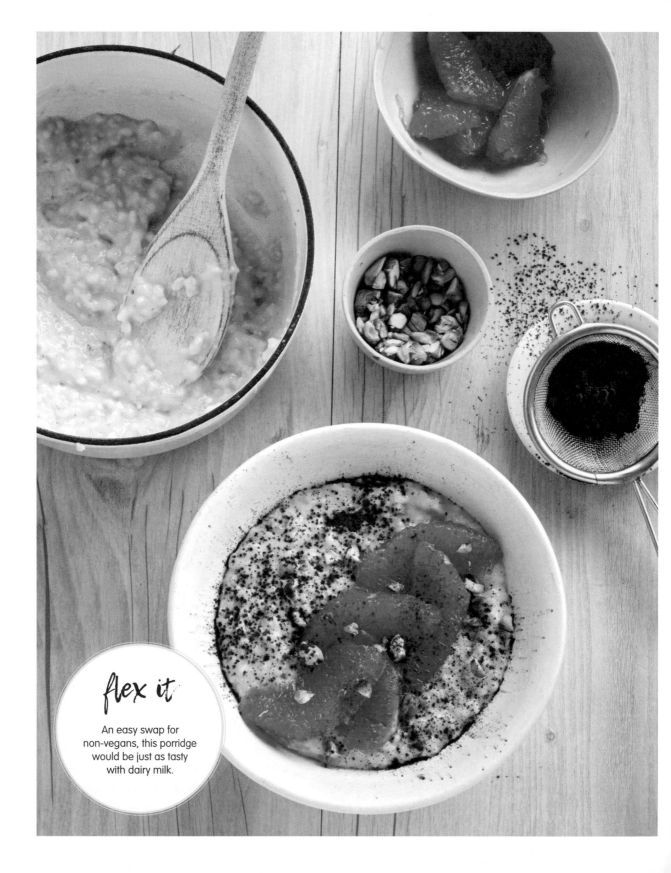

flex it

An easy swap for
non-vegans, this porridge
would be just as tasty
with dairy milk.

OAT & ALMOND MILK PORRIDGE
with grapefruit & cocoa

SERVES 2
PREP 5 MINS
COOK 15 MINS

50g (1⅔oz) **rolled oats**
240ml (8fl oz) **almond milk**
1 **pink grapefruit**, peeled and segmented
¼ tsp **vegan cocoa powder**
1 tsp **pistachio nuts**, chopped

1 Put the oats in a saucepan, then stir in the almond milk and 240ml (8fl oz) of water. Bring to the boil, then reduce the heat to a gentle simmer. Cook for 10–15 minutes, stirring occasionally, or until creamy.

2 Spoon the porridge into a serving bowl, add the grapefruit, and sprinkle over the cocoa powder and pistachio nuts.

VARIATION

For a variation, top your porridge with peach or apricot halves, a sprinkle of chopped almonds, and a drizzle of maple syrup.

the good stuff

Pistachios are full of antioxidants which help to shield the body from harmful chemicals – free radicals. Grapefruit packs a powerful nutritional punch, providing nearly half your daily vitamin C requirements.

QUINOA & BUCKWHEAT GRANOLA
with seeds & apricots

SERVES 4–6
PREP 10 MINS, plus soaking
COOK 55 MINS

150g (5½oz) **quinoa**
115g (4oz) **rolled oats**
125g (4½oz) **buckwheat groats**
85g (3oz) **sunflower seeds**
85g (3oz) **pumpkin seeds**
85g (3oz) **chia seeds**
60g (2oz) **desiccated coconut**
100g (3½oz) **walnut pieces**
1 tbsp **ground cinnamon**
100ml (3½fl oz) **maple syrup**
60g (2oz) **coconut oil**
2 tsp **vanilla extract**
100g (3½oz) **raisins**
50g (1¾oz) **dried apricots**,
  finely chopped
nut milk, to serve

1 Preheat the oven to 160°C (325°F/Gas 3). Line 2–3 large baking trays with baking parchment.

2 Put the quinoa in a sieve and rinse under cold running water. Put in a pan with 500ml (16fl oz) of water. Bring to the boil, cover, and simmer for 12 minutes or until al dente.

3 Strain and transfer to a mixing bowl. Add the oats, buckwheat, seeds, coconut, walnuts, and cinnamon.

4 In a small pan, gently heat the syrup, oil, and vanilla until combined. Stir into the quinoa mixture and leave to soak for 10 minutes.

5 Spread out 1cm (½in) thick on the trays. Bake for 20 minutes, then stir. Turn the oven down to 140°C (275°F/Gas 1) and bake for 20 minutes, then stir. Cook for 20 minutes more.

6 Combine the raisins and apricots and divide equally between the trays. Leave to cool completely before transferring to an airtight container, or serving.

the good stuff

The nuts, seeds, and grains in this granola are full of healthy fats and micronutrients. Dried apricots are rich in potassium – so adding them to your diet can help you maintain a healthy blood pressure.

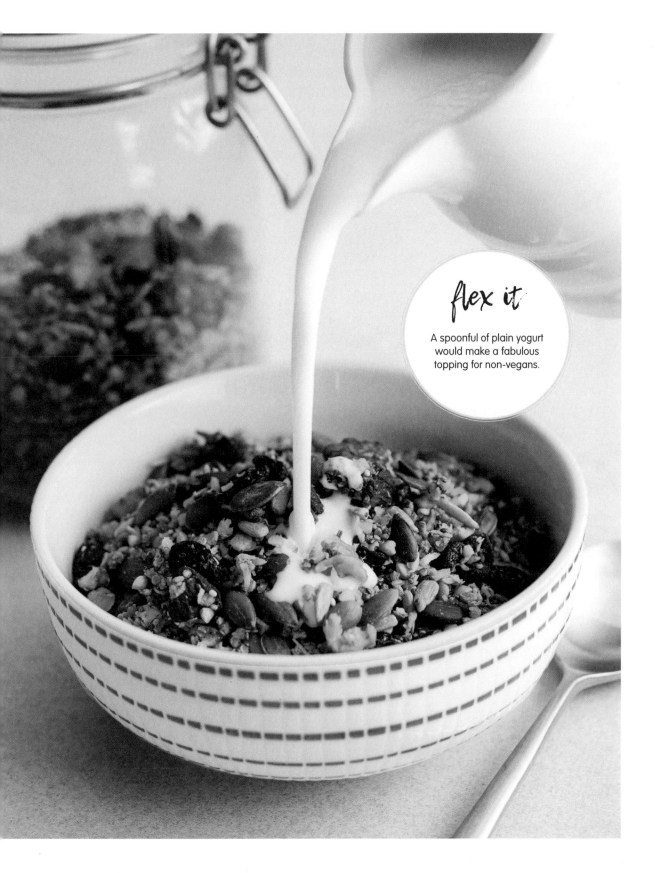

flex it

A spoonful of plain yogurt would make a fabulous topping for non-vegans.

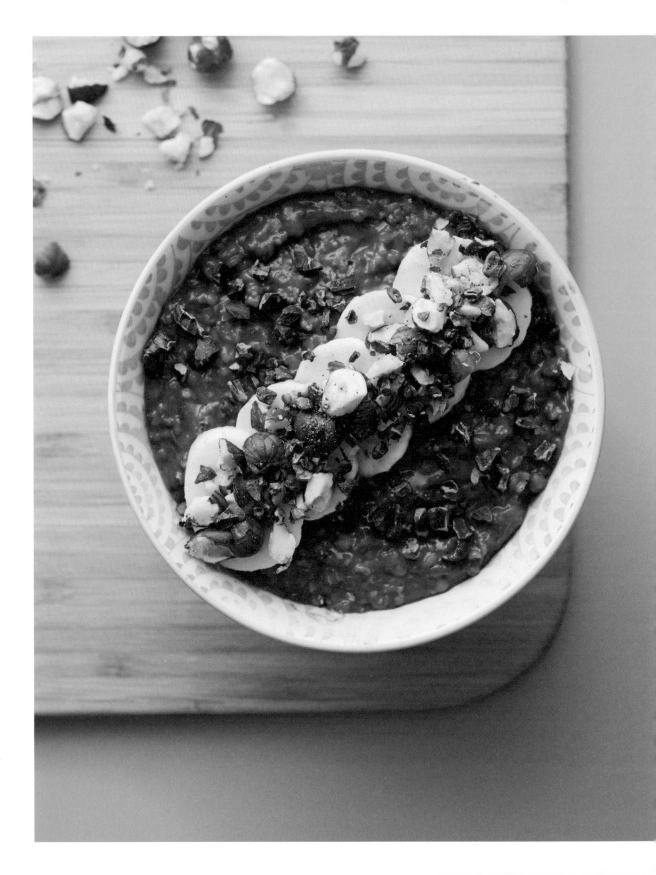

CHOCOLATE & HAZELNUT PORRIDGE
with banana & maple syrup

SERVES 2
PREP 5 MINS,
 plus soaking
COOK 20 MINS

60g (2oz) **rolled oats**
350ml (11fl oz) **hazelnut milk**
75g (2½oz) **banana**, sliced
2 tbsp **maple syrup**
1 tbsp **raw cacao powder**
1 tbsp **hazelnuts**, crushed

TOPPING
1 tbsp **hazelnuts**, crushed
1 tbsp **cacao nibs**, crushed
½ **banana**, sliced
maple syrup, to taste (optional)

1 Put the oats, hazelnut milk, banana, maple syrup, cacao powder, and hazelnuts in a saucepan over a medium heat. Bring to the boil, stirring all the time with a wooden spoon.

2 Lower the heat and simmer for 5 minutes, stirring often, until the porridge is the consistency you like (add more hazelnut milk, if you want it a little runnier).

3 Transfer to bowls and serve straightaway, sprinkled with the topping ingredients, and drizzled with more maple syrup, if you like.

the good stuff

Oats are a good source of slow-releasing energy and packed with iron. Cacao is a healthy "chocolate" option for vegans. It is supercharged with magnesium, calcium, iron, and zinc.

ANCIENT GRAINS PORRIDGE WITH PEAR
topped with pistachio & pomegranate seeds

SERVES 1
PREP 10 MINS, plus soaking
COOK 15 MINS

1 tbsp **millet**
1 tbsp **amaranth**
1 tbsp **buckwheat groats**
1 tbsp **quinoa**
200ml (7fl oz) **almond milk**, plus
    extra if desired
1 small ripe **pear**, peeled
    and cored
1 tbsp **pomegranate seeds**
1 tbsp **pistachio nuts**, crushed
1 tbsp **plant-based cream**
pinch of **ground cinnamon**
maple syrup, to taste

1 Combine the grains and soak overnight in double the volume of water. In the morning, drain and rinse well.

2 Place the grains in a saucepan with the almond milk. Bring to the boil, then turn down the heat and simmer gently for 15 minutes, stirring occasionally, until most of the almond milk is absorbed and the grains are soft – these grains have more texture and "bite" than oats.

3 Add some more almond milk if you like your porridge a little runnier.

4 Roughly mash half the pear with a fork and stir through the porridge. Cut the remaining pear into chunks.

5 Place the porridge in a bowl and top with the chunks of pear, pomegranate seeds, pistachio nuts, a drizzle of the cream, and a pinch of cinnamon.

6 Sweeten with maple syrup to taste.

the good stuff

Pears contain plenty of fibre, so are a good breakfast choice to help kick-start the digestive system. Pomegranate seeds contain high levels of antioxidants and vitamin B5, which helps you convert the food you eat into energy.

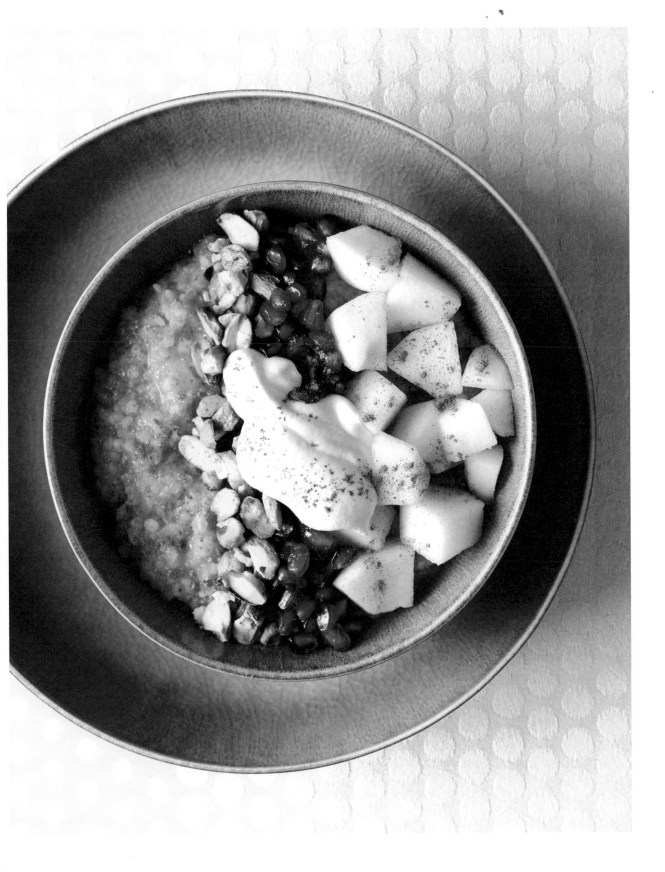

BREAKFAST BURRITOS
with mushrooms & black beans

SERVES 2
PREP 10 MINS
COOK 10 MINS

2 tbsp **olive oil**
½ small **red onion**, thinly sliced
140g (5oz) **button mushrooms**,
   sliced
1 tsp crumbled **dried sage**
½ tsp **sea salt**
½ tsp freshly ground **black pepper**
60g (2oz) cooked **black beans**
2 x 25cm (10in) **wholewheat
   tortillas**
1 large **tomato**, diced
1 **avocado**, sliced
4 tbsp shop bought **salsa**

1 Heat the olive oil in a medium sauté pan over a medium–high heat. Add the onion and mushrooms, and cook for 2–3 minutes, stirring once or twice.

2 Add the sage, salt, and black pepper, and cook for 2 more minutes.

3 Stir in the black beans and cook, turning a few times and pressing to break up the beans and brown them a little, for about 5 minutes. Remove from the heat, and set aside.

4 Lay each tortilla on a plate, and spoon half of the mushroom filling down the centre of each, and divide the tomato, avocado, and salsa between each burrito. Roll the burritos by folding two sides in first and then folding one long side inwards.

the good stuff

Black beans make a healthy addition to a vegan diet as they are high in protein with trace amounts of saturated fat and no cholesterol. They are also a great plant-based source of iron.

WHOLEWHEAT BANANA PECAN PANCAKES
with fresh mixed berries

MAKES 12
PREP 15 MINS
COOK 10 MINS

300ml (10fl oz) **soya milk** or
  coconut milk, plus extra
  if needed
1 tbsp **ground flax seeds**
1 tsp **apple cider vinegar**
1 large ripe **banana**, peeled and
  mashed well
1 tbsp **brown sugar**
1 tbsp **maple syrup**, plus more for
  serving (optional)
1 tsp **vanilla extract**
120g (4oz) **wholemeal flour**
45g (1½oz) **buckwheat flour**
2 tsp **baking powder**
½ tsp **sea salt**
½ tsp **ground cinnamon**
¼ tsp **ground nutmeg**
75g (2½oz) **pecan nuts**, toasted
  and finely chopped
150g (5¼oz) mixed **raspberries,
blueberries**, and/or **strawberries**
(optional)

1. Warm 60ml (2fl oz) of the soya or coconut milk in a small pan over a medium–high heat.

2. Place the ground flax seeds in a bowl, add the warmed milk, stir well, and set aside.

3. In a small bowl, whisk the apple cider vinegar into the remaining soya milk, and set aside to thicken and curdle.

4. In another small bowl, mash the banana with the brown sugar, maple syrup, and vanilla extract. Whisk in the flax mixture, followed by the curdled soya milk, and blend well.

5. Heat a cast-iron griddle or frying pan over a medium heat until a drop of water sizzles and evaporates immediately.

6. Meanwhile, in a medium bowl, whisk together the wholemeal flour, buckwheat flour, baking powder, salt, cinnamon, and nutmeg. Stir in the wet ingredients until just combined, and quickly fold in the chopped pecans. Stir in more soya milk, as needed, to make a thick batter; you want it to be the consistency of a heavy cake mixture.

7. Lightly oil or butter the griddle, and drop 3 tablespoon-size scoops of batter into the pan, spreading with a small spatula if necessary. Cook for 2 minutes without disturbing or until bubbles form on the surface of the pancakes, carefully flip over the pancakes, and cook for a further 1½ minutes. Grease the pan a little between each batch, as these pancakes may stick otherwise.

8. Serve hot with mixed fruit (if using) and more maple syrup (if using).

SNACKS & LIGHT BITES

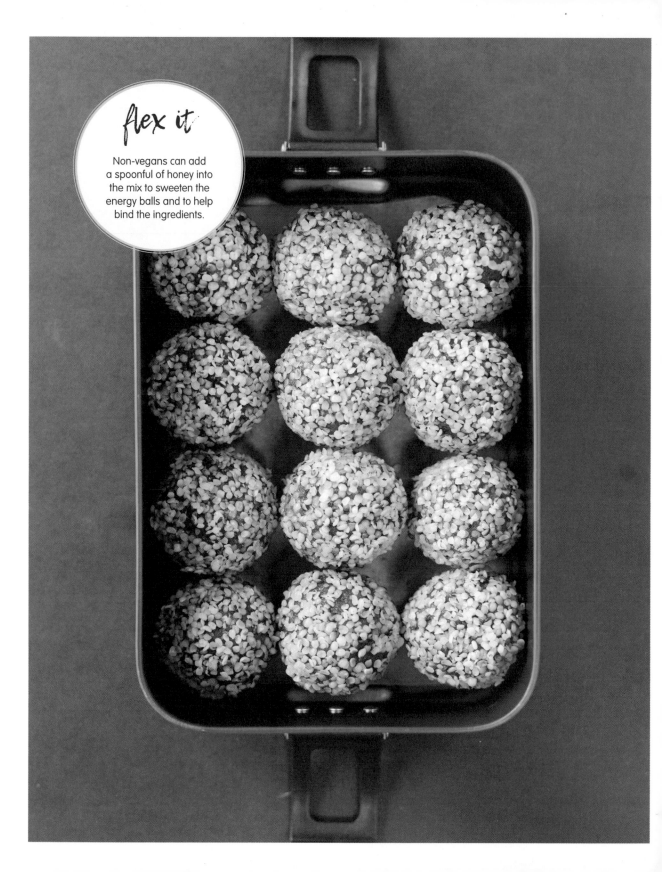

flex it

Non-vegans can add a spoonful of honey into the mix to sweeten the energy balls and to help bind the ingredients.

PEANUT BUTTER & BANANA BALLS
with dates & hemp seeds

MAKES 16
PREP 20 MINS, plus chilling

140g (5oz) **unsalted crunchy peanut butter**
1 small ripe **banana** (about 75g/2½oz)
140g (5oz) **dates**
30g (1oz) **ground flax seeds**
30g (1oz) **chia seeds**
20g (¾oz) **ground almonds**
2 tsp **moringa powder**, to taste
shelled hemp seeds, to coat

1 Place all the ingredients except the hemp seeds in a food processor and pulse until the mixture starts to come together, forming a loose ball.

2 Divide into 16 evenly sized portions and roll into balls.

3 Sprinkle a layer of hemp seeds on a separate plate and gently roll the balls to coat.

4 Place in the fridge for 1 hour or in the freezer for 20 minutes to firm up before eating. Best served chilled.

the good stuff

A sugar-free peanut butter is a good energy source for a mid-morning snack. These balls also contain moringa powder, a nutrient-dense leaf with a spinachy taste. Chia seeds are rich in fibre, omega-3 fats, protein, vitamins and minerals.

AVOCADO & BANANA RECOVERY ICE BITES
with cacao & chia seeds

MAKES 8
PREP 10 MINS, plus chilling
COOK 5 MINS

400ml (14fl oz) **unsweetened almond** or **hazelnut milk**
2 tbsp **cacao nibs**
1 tbsp **chia seeds**
½ ripe **avocado**
1 small **banana**
pinch of **sea salt**

1 Pour the almond or hazelnut milk into a small pan and sprinkle in the cacao nibs. Warm gently, bring to a simmer, then remove from the heat. Leave to cool slightly, stir in the chia seeds, then leave to cool completely.

2 Tip the avocado and banana into the bowl of a food processor and blend well with a pinch of salt. Add the cooled milk mixture to the bowl and whizz again, to break up the cacao nibs a little but not so that they are smooth.

3 Using a small plastic funnel or a funnel made from parchment paper, pour the mixture into eight 60ml (2fl oz) spherical ice lolly moulds. Alternatively, try ice-lolly moulds or large ice-cube trays. Place in the freezer.

4 When the bites are half-frozen, insert a lolly stick or cake pop stick into each one. Return to the freezer and freeze until hard.

the good stuff

Avocados are loaded with good fats and they are a good source of B vitamins. What's more, you are getting a double amount of potassium by eating avocado and banana. Adding a serving of chia seeds a day to your diet can help boost your metabolism.

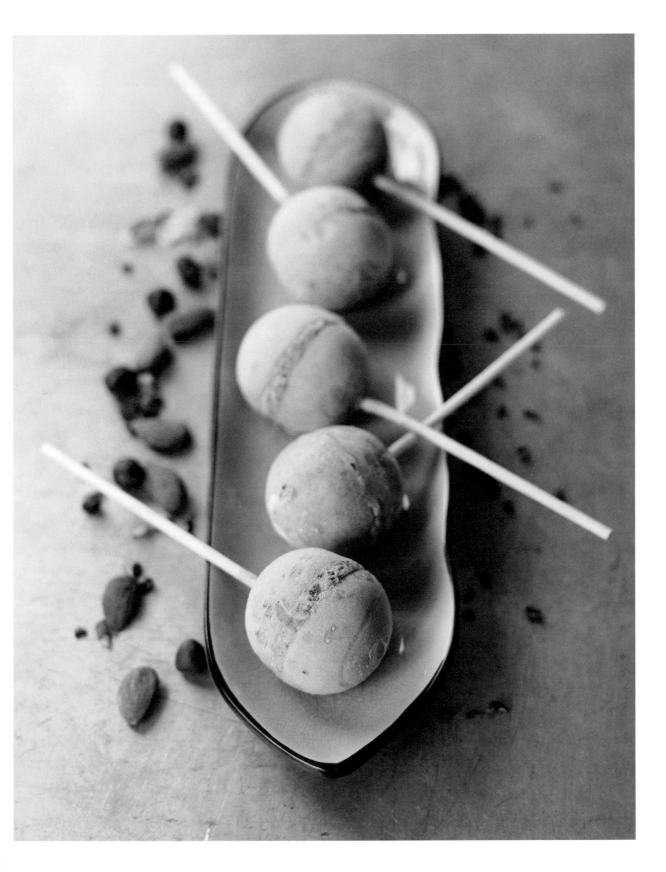

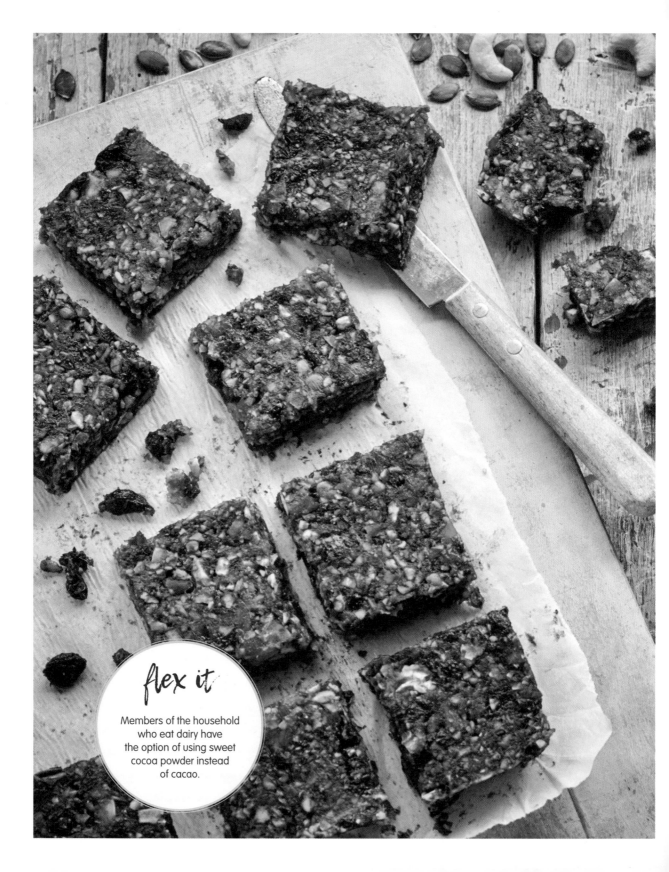

flex it

Members of the household who eat dairy have the option of using sweet cocoa powder instead of cacao.

RAW ENERGY BARS
with dates & dried apricots

MAKES 16
PREP 20 MINS, plus chilling

200g (7oz) **Medjool dates**,
  pitted and roughly chopped
115g (4oz) **dried apricots**,
  roughly chopped
60g (2oz) **dried cherries**
or **cranberries**, roughly chopped
60g (2oz) **flaked almonds**
60g (2oz) **cashew nuts**,
  roughly chopped
30g (1oz) **pumpkin seeds**
30g (1oz) **sunflower seeds**
30g (1oz) **flaked coconut**
2 tbsp **raw cacao powder**

1 Line a 20cm (8in) square baking tray with baking parchment. Place the chopped dates in a heatproof bowl and cover with hot water. Leave them to soak while you prepare the rest of the ingredients.

2 After 5 minutes, drain the dates using a sieve. When cool enough to handle, press the dates lightly to remove some of the water, leaving them just a little damp. Place them in a food processor and add all the remaining ingredients.

3 Process the mixture until it is well combined, the nuts and seeds are in small pieces, and the mixture begins to form a ball in the bowl of the food processor. If the mixture is not blending thoroughly, take some out and process it in batches.

4 Dampen your hands and turn the mixture out into the lined baking tray. Push the mixture into an even layer using your hands. Dampen the back of a large metal spoon, and use it to even out the surface of the mixture. Place the filled tray in the fridge for 3–4 hours.

5 Turn the mixture out onto a board and cut into 16 squares. Wrap the squares individually in greaseproof paper to prevent them from sticking together, and store in an airtight container in the fridge until needed.

the good stuff

These no-bake bars combine fibre-rich dried fruit with protein-rich nuts and seeds. They are perfect to eat on the go as part of a plant-based diet, as they will provide bags of energy.

NUT & SEED NUTRIENT BOOSTERS
with chickpeas & lentils

MAKES 16
PREP 30 MINS, plus soaking
COOK 1 HR 20 MINS

60g (2oz) **chickpeas**, soaked
  overnight
30g (1oz) **brown rice**
100g (3½oz) **red split lentils**
75g (2½oz) **broccoli**, chopped
½ **red pepper**, deseeded
  and finely chopped
1 **celery stick**, finely chopped
25g (1oz) **pumpkin seeds**
25g (1oz) **sunflower seeds**
1 tsp **thyme leaves**
85g (3oz) **cashew nuts**
50g (1¾oz) whole **almonds**
½ tsp **tamari**
1 tsp **brown miso paste**
sesame or **chia seeds**,
  to coat (optional)

1 Drain the soaked chickpeas and rinse under cold water. Place in a pan with 300ml (10fl oz) of boiling, salted water. Bring back to the boil, cover, and simmer for 1 hour until the chickpeas are soft, but not soggy – they should have some "bite". Drain and put to one side.

2 Bring the rice to the boil in salted water, then simmer for about 30 minutes until really soft. Drain and put to one side.

3 Rinse the lentils under cold water. Place in a pan with 300ml (10fl oz) of boiling, salted water. Bring back to the boil, cover, and simmer for 10 minutes until the lentils are soft, but not soggy. Drain and put to one side.

4 Combine the rice, lentils, broccoli, pepper, celery, seeds, and thyme in a large bowl.

5 Put the chickpeas, nuts, tamari, and miso in a food processor and whizz until you have a rough paste. – you don't want a purée. Add this mixture to the rice bowl, combine well and season.

6 Preheat the oven to 180°C (400°F/Gas 6). Line a large baking tray with baking parchment. Divide the mixture into 16 evenly sized portions and roll into balls. If you wish, roll the balls in sesame seeds and/or chia seeds, to coat them. Place on the baking tray.

7 Bake in the preheated oven for 20 minutes until golden brown. Remove and leave to cool on a wire rack for a few minutes before serving hot. Alternatively, serve cold.

the good stuff

Due to the chickpeas and lentils, these powerful little bites are high in fibre and protein. This means they will boost your energy and keep you full for longer – curbing those unhealthy snack cravings. The nuts and seeds are packed with healthy fats and minerals.

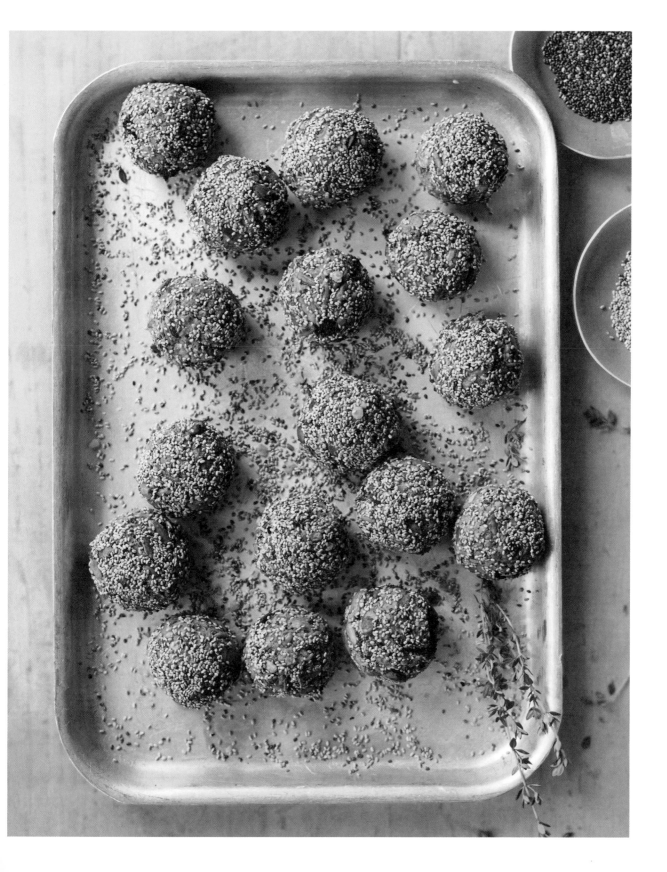

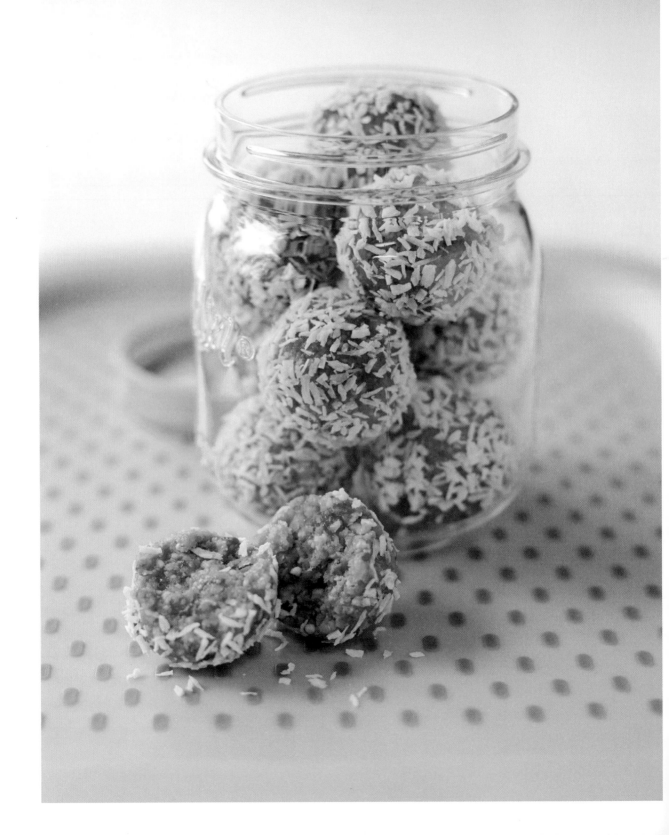

TROPICAL IMMUNE BOOSTERS
with mango & goji berries

MAKES 16
PREP 20 MINS, plus chilling

140g (5oz) **dried mango**
30g (1oz) **goji berries**
140g (5oz) **cashew nuts**
60g (2oz) **desiccated coconut**,
  plus extra to coat
1 tbsp **baobab powder**
1¼ tsp **ground turmeric**
1 tsp **rosehip powder**
juice and zest of 1 **lime**

1   Place all the ingredients in a food processor and pulse until finely chopped.

2   With the motor running, add 2–4 tablespoons of cold water a little at a time until the mixture starts to come together, forming a loose ball.

3   Divide into 16 evenly sized portions and roll into balls.

4   Sprinkle a layer of desiccated coconut on a separate plate and gently roll the balls to coat.

5   Place in the fridge for 1 hour or freeze for 20 minutes to firm up before eating. Best served chilled, but fine popped in a lunchbox and eaten later in the day.

the good stuff

Turmeric is an anti-inflammatory; introducing it into the diet can help protect against colds and flu. Goji berries pack a punch for their size – they are full of vitamins A and C, iron, potassium, and calcium.

LEMONY SPINACH HUMMUS
with tahini & chia seeds

SERVES 6
PREP 5 MINS

150g (5½oz) cooked **chickpeas**,
   peeled
75g (2½oz) **baby spinach**
2 **garlic cloves**
juice and zest of 1 large **lemon**
1 tbsp **tahini**
60ml (2fl oz) **olive oil**
salt and freshly ground
   black pepper
1½ tbsp **chia seeds**,
   to garnish
alfalfa sprouts, to garnish
microgreens, to garnish

1 In a food processor, combine the chickpeas, spinach, garlic, lemon juice and zest, and tahini. Process on low for 1 minute to combine the ingredients.

2 With the processor on high, drizzle in the oil. For a thinner consistency, gradually add cold water, 1 tablespoon at a time, until the desired texture is achieved. Add salt and pepper to taste.

3 Transfer to a serving bowl and garnish with chia seeds, sprouts, and microgreens. Serve immediately.

the good stuff

Leafy green spinach is a must for a vegan diet, as it is packed with vitamins K, A, C, B6, B12, and E. Vitamins C, E, and A are particularly good for your skin, cleansing it from the inside out.

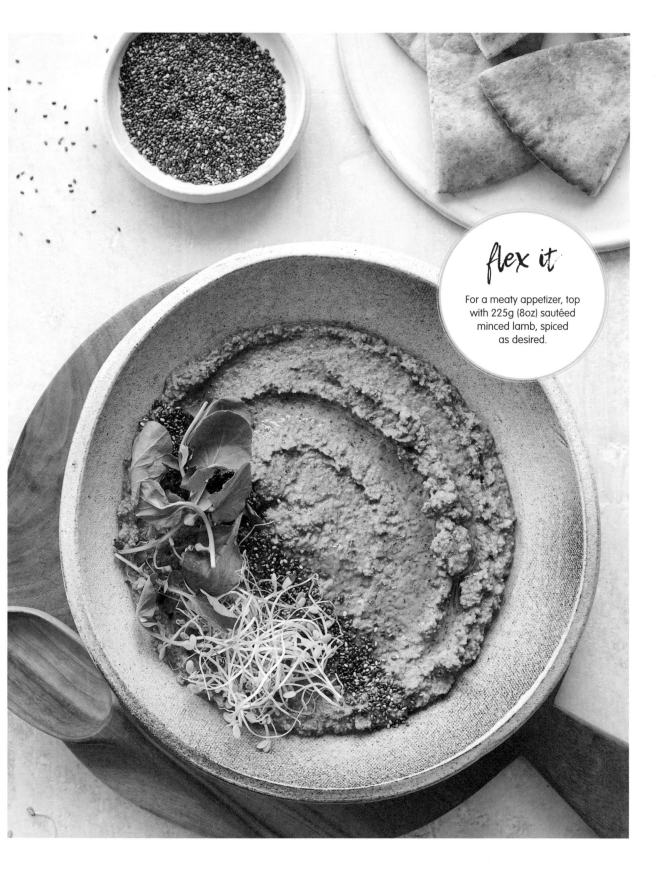

flex it

For a meaty appetizer, top with 225g (8oz) sautéed minced lamb, spiced as desired.

CASHEW RICOTTA
with parsley & chives

SERVES 8
PREP 10 MINS, plus soaking

280g (9½oz) **cashew nuts**

4 tbsp **extra virgin olive oil**

juice of 1½ **lemons**

2 tbsp **nutritional yeast**

1 tbsp finely chopped **parsley**

1 tbsp finely chopped **chives**

1 tsp **white (shiro) miso**

½ tsp **dried marjoram**

½ tsp **sea salt**

½ tsp freshly ground **black pepper**

1 Soak the cashew nuts in water overnight.

2 Discard the soaking water, rinse the cashews well, and drain.

3 In a food processor fitted with a metal blade, process the cashews along with the olive oil, 4 tablespoons of warm water, the lemon juice, nutritional yeast, parsley, chives, miso, marjoram, salt, and black pepper until smooth.

4 Spread this nutty "cheese" on crackers or use it as a filling for ravioli or lasagne. You can store it in the fridge for up to 5 days.

CHICKPEA BITES
with peanut butter

MAKES 24
PREP 15 MINS, plus chilling

350g (12oz) cooked **chickpeas**

125g (4½oz) **smooth peanut butter**

45g (1½oz) **rolled oats**

80ml (3fl oz) **agave nectar**

1 tsp **vanilla extract**

1 tsp **ground cinnamon**

pinch of **salt**

1 In a food processor, pulse the chickpeas until coarsely ground. Transfer to a large mixing bowl. Stir in the peanut butter, oats, agave, vanilla extract, cinnamon, and salt.

2 Take 1 heaped tablespoon of the chickpea mixture and roll into a ball with your hands. Repeat with the remaining chickpea mixture to make 24 in total. Chill to set in an airtight container in the fridge for at least 1 hour, or overnight, before serving.

the good stuff

Chickpeas are packed with essential micronutrients. Oats are full of magnesium, which can help with moods. They also have a high fibre content, keeping you fuller for longer, which makes them the perfect snack food.

POLENTA FRIES
with rosemary & garlic

SERVES 4–6
PREP 15 MINS, plus chilling
COOK 30 MINS

1–2 tbsp **olive oil**,
  plus extra for greasing
750ml (1¼ pints) **vegetable stock**
1 tbsp **plant-based margarine**
150g (5½oz) **quick-cook polenta**
1 **garlic clove**, pressed
1 tbsp finely chopped **rosemary**
salt and freshly ground
  black pepper

1 Grease a baking sheet and set aside. Place the stock and margarine in a saucepan and bring to the boil. Then reduce the heat to medium–low and gradually add the polenta, whisking constantly. Cook for about 2 minutes, whisking constantly, until all the liquid has been absorbed and the polenta has thickened and is smooth.

2 Remove from the heat, add the garlic and rosemary, and mix well to combine. Transfer the polenta mixture to the baking sheet and spread it out to form an even 1cm (½in) thick layer. Place the baking sheet in the refrigerator to chill for 3 hours.

3 Preheat the oven to 200°C (400°F/Gas 6). Grease another baking sheet and set aside. Place the polenta on a clean surface and slice into long rectangular pieces. Spread out the fries on the prepared baking sheet and lightly brush with oil. Season well and bake for 20–25 minutes or until they are golden brown at the edges. Remove from the heat and serve immediately.

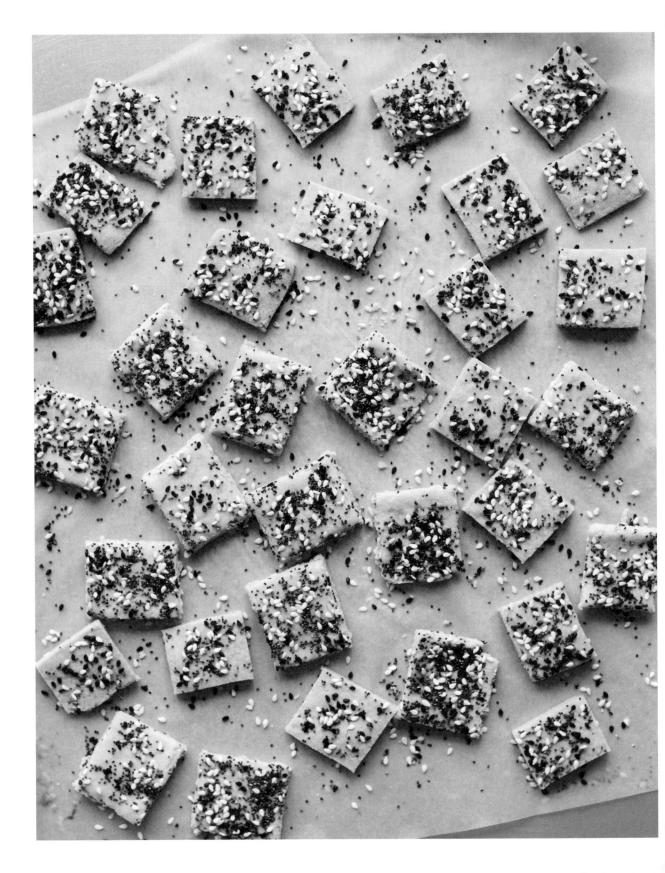

GARLICKY ONION CRACKERS
with a trio of seeds

MAKES 24
PREP 30 MINS
COOK 15 MINS

½ tbsp **sesame seeds**
½ tbsp **black sesame seeds**
½ tbsp **poppy seeds**
½ tsp **baking powder**
115g (4oz) **chickpea flour**
¾ tsp **salt**
⅛ tsp **onion powder**
⅛ tsp **garlic powder**
2 tbsp **olive oil**

1 To make the topping, in a small bowl combine the sesame seeds, black sesame seeds, and poppy seeds. Set aside.

2 Preheat the oven to 190°C (375°F/Gas 5). Prepare a clean, flat work surface and cut 2 large pieces of baking parchment, each about 30 x 40cm (12 x 16in).

3 To make the dough, in a large mixing bowl combine the baking powder, chickpea flour, salt, onion powder, garlic powder, and oil. Gradually incorporate 60ml (2fl oz) of water until a dough forms, adding additional water a spoonful at a time as needed, until the dough is just pliable. Place in the fridge to rest for 10 minutes.

4 Divide the dough into 2 pieces and place side by side between the two sheets of baking parchment, about 12cm (5in) apart. With a rolling pin, roll out as thinly as possible into 2 rectangles, about 3mm (⅛in) thick.

5 Remove the top sheet of baking parchment. With a pizza cutter or paring knife, score the dough into 3 x 3cm (1 x 1in) squares, making 24 crackers. Brush the dough with 1–2 teaspoons of water, then sprinkle the seed mixture evenly across the top.

6 Transfer the bottom piece of baking parchment directly onto a baking sheet. Bake for 10–15 minutes until the edges start to brown and the crackers are firm. Leave to rest at room temperature for 5 minutes, then break the crackers apart. Store in an airtight container for up to 3 days.

MUNG BEAN GUACAMOLE
with lime & coriander

SERVES 2
PREP 20 MINS

2 large **avocados**
juice of 1 **lime**
1 **onion**, finely chopped
2 **garlic cloves**, finely chopped
1 **tomato**, diced
85g (3oz) cooked **mung beans**
2 tbsp roughly chopped
  coriander leaves
salt and freshly ground
  black pepper

1 Cut the avocados in half, remove the stones, and scoop the flesh into a large bowl. Immediately add the lime juice. With a pastry cutter or fork, roughly mash the avocado.

2 Add the onion, garlic, tomato, mung beans, and coriander. Stir gently to combine. Season with salt and pepper to taste. Serve immediately.

VARIATION

Swap the mung beans for black beans, or use a white bean such as cannellini beans. For a change, you could also stir through a few chopped green olives, some finely chopped red peppers, roasted garlic, or some toasted pumpkin seeds.

the good stuff

The addition of mung beans brings a nutritional boost and an extra creamy texture to this Mexican classic. Mung beans are an excellent source of folate, magnesium, and vitamin B1. They are also high in fibre and protein.

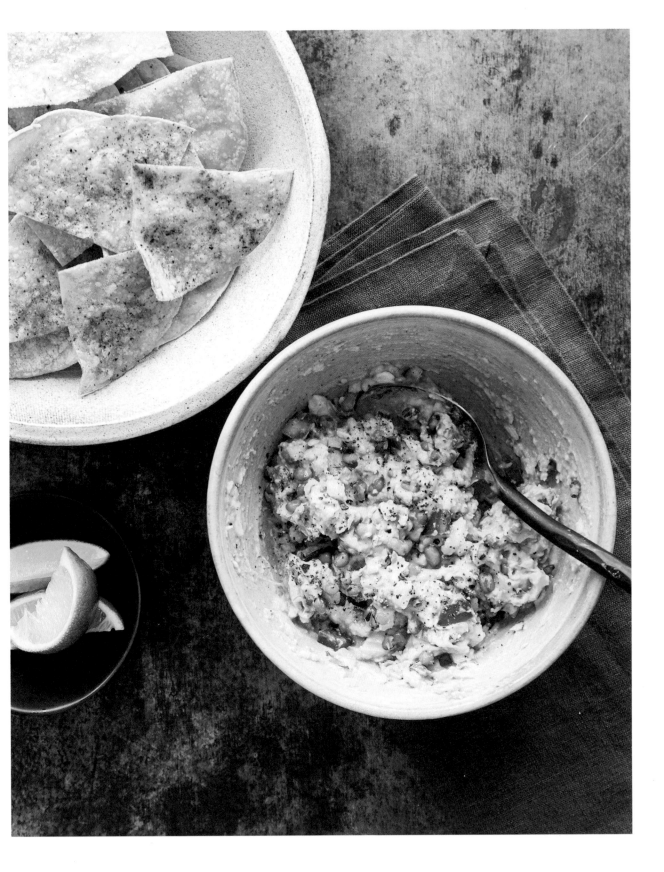

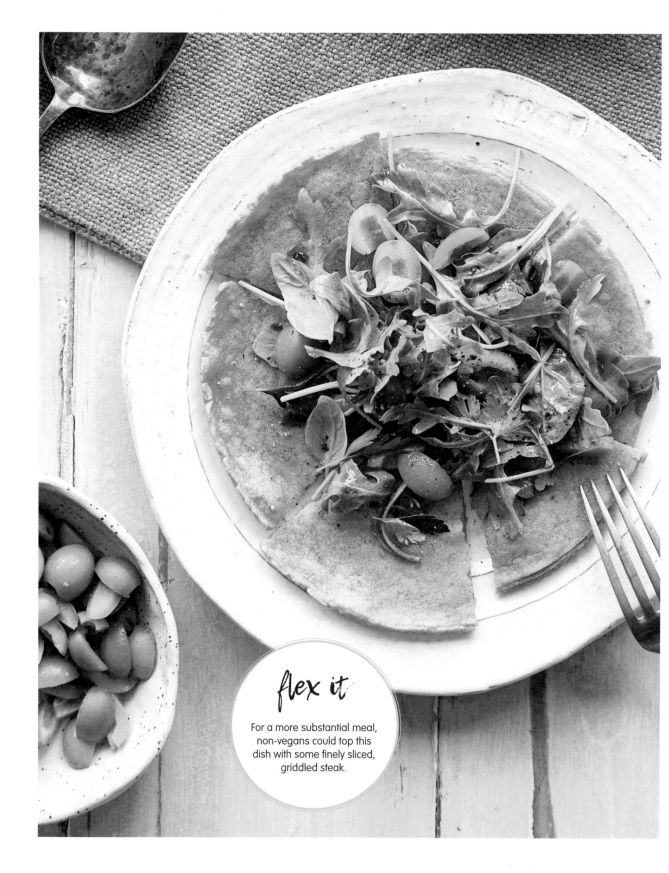

flex it

For a more substantial meal,
non-vegans could top this
dish with some finely sliced,
griddled steak.

CHICKPEA FLOUR SOCCA
with herb & green olive salad

SERVES 2
PREP 5 MINS, plus resting
COOK 15 MINS

100g (3½oz) **chickpea flour**
1 tsp **smoked paprika**
⅛ tsp **garlic powder**
pinch of **salt**
3 tbsp **olive oil**
45g (1½oz) **rocket leaves**
10g (¼oz) **flat-leaf parsley**
5g (⅛oz) **basil leaves**
45g (1½oz) **green olives**,
  pitted and halved
juice of 1 **lemon**

1 To make the batter, in a medium mixing bowl add the chickpea flour, paprika, garlic powder, salt, 2 tablespoons of the olive oil, and 240ml (8fl oz) of water. Whisk to combine. Let rest at room temperature for 1 hour.

2 With the rack in the middle of the oven, place two 20cm (8in) cast-iron or ovenproof frying pans in the oven and preheat to the highest setting. (The pans will heat up with the oven.)

3 When the frying pans are heated, carefully remove and swirl 1½ teaspoons of oil around in each. Pour half the batter into each and return to the oven. Bake for 8 minutes. Then turn the grill onto a low setting and cook for an additional 2 minutes. Remove and let rest for 1–2 minutes.

4 Meanwhile, to make the herb and olive salad, toss together the rocket, parsley, basil, olives, and lemon juice. Place each socca on a serving plate and top with an equal amount of salad. Serve immediately.

the good stuff

Chickpea flour, also know as gram flour, is naturally gluten-free. It adds a nutty taste and boost of protein, and is an excellent source of folate, necessary for supporting immune functions.

SPROUTED SUMMER ROLLS
with chilli-lime dipping sauce

MAKES 8
PREP 20 MINS

30g (1oz) **bean thread** (cellophane)
   noodles
8 × 15cm (6in) diameter **rice
   paper wrappers**
1 **carrot**, peeled, and julienned into
   5cm (2in) pieces
5cm (2in) piece of **cucumber**,
   quartered, deseeded, and
   julienned
handful of **radish sprouts**
handful of **mustard sprouts**
15g (½oz) **pea shoots**
large handful of mixed **mint**,
   coriander, and **Thai basil leaves**,
   roughly chopped

DIPPING SAUCE
½ mild **red chilli**, finely chopped
½ **garlic clove**, very finely sliced
2 tbsp **rice wine vinegar**
1 tbsp **lime juice**
1 tbsp **sugar**
1 tsp fine **sea salt**

1   To make the dipping sauce, whisk together the chilli, garlic, vinegar, lime juice, sugar, and salt with 3 tablespoons of warm water. Set aside.

2   To prepare the noodles, place in a bowl and cover with just-boiled water. Let sit for 5 minutes, then drain and dry well.

3   Soak 1 rice paper wrapper in a bowl of warm water for 10–15 seconds. Once soft, place the wrapper on a clean, damp tea towel. On the lower one-third of the paper, make a rectangular pile of 1 tablespoon of the noodles and equal quantities of the vegetables, sprouts, and shoots, leaving a 1cm (½in) border on each side. Top with a sprinkle of the herbs.

4   Lift the lower edge of the rice paper and fold it over the filling. Tightly tuck the sides in and over the edges of the filling, then roll up the summer roll, keeping the filling tucked in.

5   Place the roll seam-side down on a serving plate and cover with a second clean, damp tea towel. Continue to make the rolls until all the filling is used up. When you have made the last roll, serve immediately with the dipping sauce alongside.

the good stuff

Radish sprouts and mustard sprouts are super nutritious as they are full of vitamin B6, a metabolism-boosting nutrient essential to include in a vegan diet. Raw sprouted seeds carry a risk of foodborne bacteria so avoid serving to children and pregnant women.

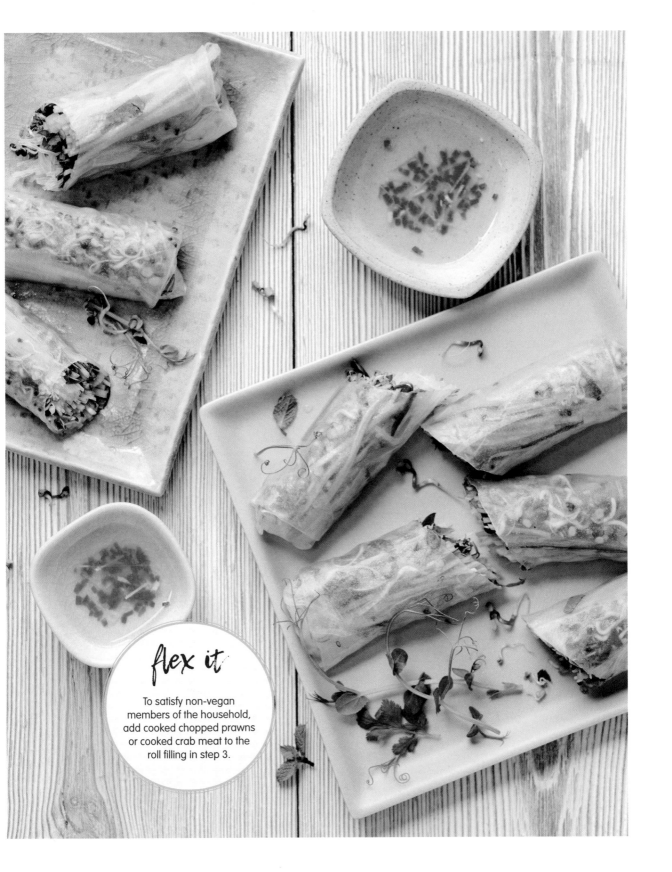

flex it

To satisfy non-vegan
members of the household,
add cooked chopped prawns
or cooked crab meat to the
roll filling in step 3.

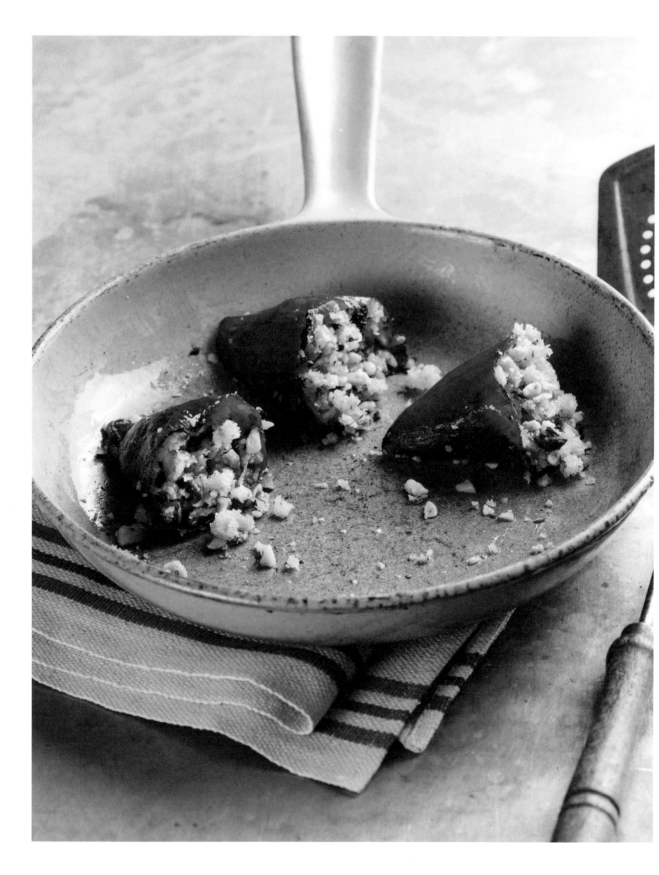

ALMOND & BREADCRUMB STUFFED PEPPERS
with chilli & capers

SERVES 4
PREP 10 MINS
COOK 30 MINS

3 tbsp **extra virgin olive oil**
2 **garlic cloves**, finely chopped
1 small **shallot**, finely chopped
½ tsp crushed **chillies**
2 tbsp finely chopped
   flat-leaf parsley
60g (2oz) fresh **breadcrumbs**
75g (2½oz) **Marcona almonds**,
   finely chopped
1 tbsp **salted capers**, rinsed,
   drained, and finely chopped
400g (14oz) can whole **piquillo**
   peppers, drained

1 Preheat the oven to 180°C (350°F/Gas 4). Heat 1 tablespoon of the olive oil in a small saucepan over a medium–high heat. Add the garlic, shallot, and crushed chillies, and cook for 30 seconds. Stir in the flat-leaf parsley and remove from the heat.

2 In a small bowl, combine the breadcrumbs, almonds, capers, and garlic mixture. Stir in 1 tablespoon of the olive oil.

3 Drizzle a medium baking dish with half of the remaining olive oil. Gently fill each piquillo pepper with about 1 tablespoon of the stuffing, and place the filled peppers in the baking dish. Drizzle the stuffed peppers with the remaining olive oil and bake for 20 minutes. Serve hot, warm, or at room temperature.

the good stuff

Garlic is an excellent source of B6, it also contains manganese, selenium, and vitamin C. Almonds are the healthiest of all the nuts and make a good ingredient to add to snack food. They are rich in vitamin E, calcium, and potassium.

ARANCINI (RISOTTO BALLS)
with panko breadcrumbs

SERVES 4
PREP 30 MINS, plus chilling
COOK 10 MINS

125g (4½oz) **plain flour**
175g (6oz) **panko breadcrumbs**
400g (14oz) of your favourite
   left over **risotto**, chilled overnight
10 x 1cm (½in) cubes **plant-based**
   mozzarella cheese
40g (1½oz) **frozen peas**
grapeseed oil, for frying
fresh tomato sauce, to serve

1 Line 2 baking sheets with baking parchment.

2 Place the flour, 120ml (4fl oz) of water, and breadcrumbs in separate small, shallow bowls.

3 Scoop out portions (each about 120ml (4fl oz/about half a mug) of chilled risotto. Using wet hands, form each portion into a ball, tucking 1 plant-based mozzarella cheese cube and a few peas into the centre. Place the balls on one of the baking sheets.

4 Working one at a time, quickly roll each ball in the flour, dip in water, and roll in the panko breadcrumbs, being sure to thoroughly coat each ball. Roll once more in the flour, shake off the excess, and set aside on the second baking sheet. When all balls are breaded, chill for 30 minutes or overnight.

5 Just before you're ready to serve, preheat the oven to 130°C (250°F/Gas ½).

6 Heat 7.5–10cm (3–4in) of grapeseed oil in a wide saucepan over a medium–high heat. Use a deep-frying thermometer to bring the oil to 190°C (375°F) and add balls, 3 or 4 at a time. Cook, turning frequently, for about 3 minutes or until golden brown all over. Transfer to a wire rack set over a baking tray to keep the balls crisp and keep warm in the oven as you fry subsequent batches. Serve hot with a fresh tomato sauce for dipping.

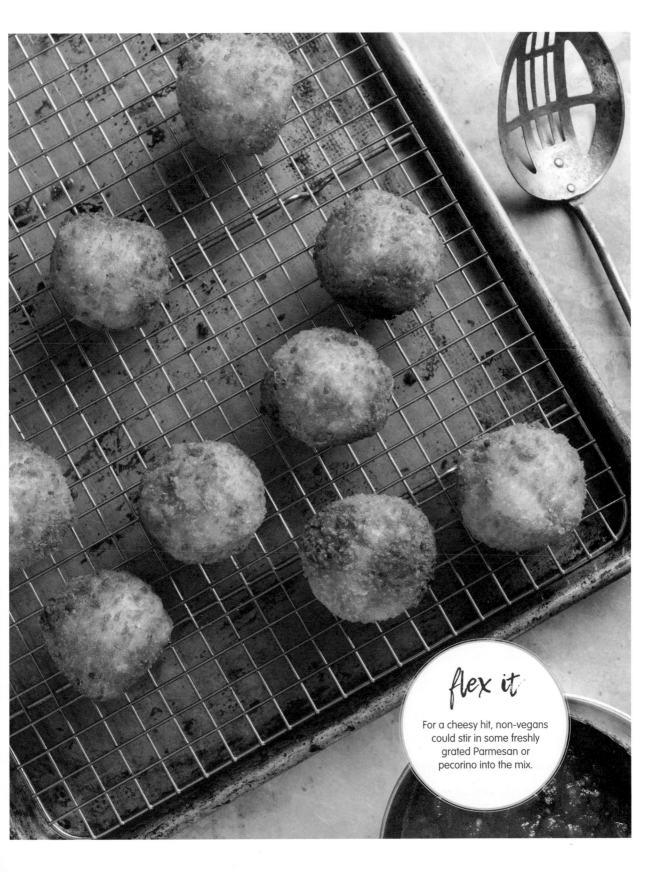

flex it

For a cheesy hit, non-vegans could stir in some freshly grated Parmesan or pecorino into the mix.

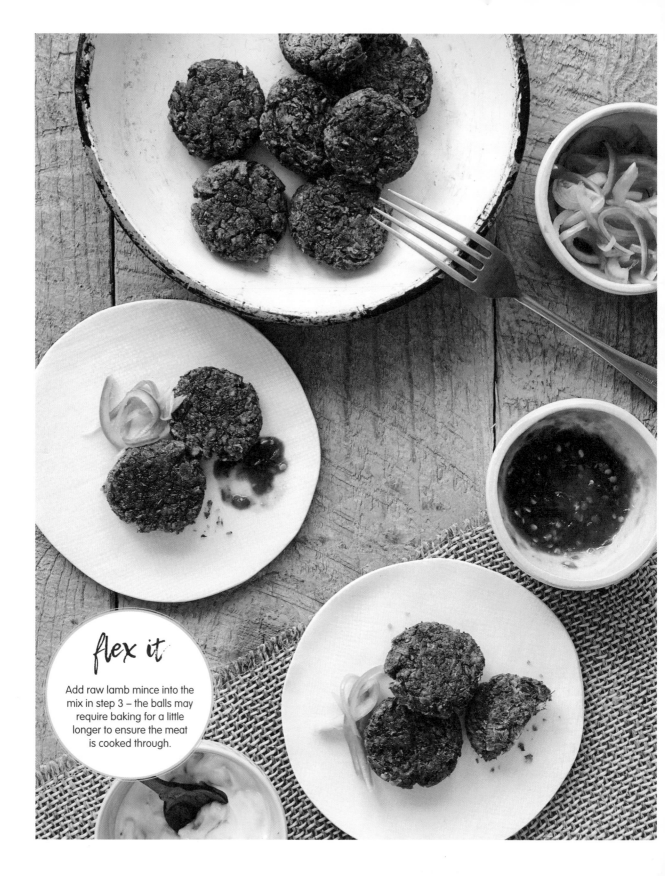

flex it

Add raw lamb mince into the mix in step 3 – the balls may require baking for a little longer to ensure the meat is cooked through.

BAKED FALAFEL
with pickled red onions & sambal oelek

MAKES 16
PREP 30 MINS, plus chilling
COOK 40 MINS

1 **garlic clove**
350g (12oz) cooked **chickpeas**
½ tsp **bicarbonate of soda**
½ tsp **ground coriander**
½ tsp **ground cumin**
pinch of crushed **dried chillies**
bunch of **curly parsley**, chopped
20g (¾oz) finely chopped **coriander leaves**
juice and zest of 1 **lemon**
20g (¾oz) **chickpea flour**
1 tbsp **olive oil**
salt and freshly ground **black pepper**
75g (2½oz) **sambal oelek**, to serve

PICKLED RED ONIONS
240ml (8fl oz) **apple cider vinegar**
120ml (4fl oz) **red wine vinegar**
2 tbsp **sugar**
1 tsp **salt**
1 large **red onion**, thinly sliced

1. To make the pickled red onions, in a medium saucepan bring the apple cider vinegar, red wine vinegar, sugar, and salt to the boil over a medium heat. Stir until the sugar and salt dissolve. Remove from the heat and stir in the red onion. Leave to cool completely at room temperature, stirring occasionally. Pour into a glass jar and secure with a lid. Refrigerate for 3 hours or overnight.

2. Preheat the oven to 200°C (400°F/Gas 6). In a food processor, combine the garlic, chickpeas, bicarbonate of soda, ground coriander, cumin, chillies, parsley, chopped coriander, and lemon zest and juice. Pulse until combined but not smooth.

3. Transfer the chickpea mixture to a medium mixing bowl and fold in the chickpea flour. Drizzle the oil over and stir once more until it holds together. Season with salt and pepper to taste.

4. Portion out approximately 2 tablespoons of chickpea mixture and roll into a ball with your hands. Place on a baking tray and repeat with the remaining mixture. With a spatula, slightly flatten each one. Bake for 10 minutes, turn over, and bake for an additional 10 minutes. Serve immediately with the pickled red onions and sambal oelek on the side.

the good stuff

For a healthier version of falafel, these are baked instead of deep-fried. With chickpeas as the base, they are also full of protein and are super filling.

SEITAN SATAY
with tamarind peanut sauce

SERVES 4
PREP 5 MINS, plus chilling
COOK 10 MINS

300g **seitan**, cut into 2.5cm (1in) chunks

8 **bamboo skewers**

6 tbsp **reduced-sodium tamari**

1 tbsp **toasted sesame oil**

1 tbsp melted **coconut oil**

3 tbsp grated **fresh root ginger**

2 **garlic cloves**, finely chopped

2 tbsp **tamarind paste**

125g (4½oz) **crunchy peanut butter**

120ml (4fl oz) **full-fat coconut milk**, well shaken

1 tsp crushed **chillies**

1 Place the seitan chunks in a baking dish large enough to hold them in a single layer.

2 In a small bowl, whisk together 4 tablespoons of the tamari, 4 tablespoons of water, the sesame oil, coconut oil, 1 tablespoon of the ginger, and garlic. Pour over the seitan, and stir well. Cover and refrigerate for 2 hours or overnight.

3 Soak 8 bamboo skewers in warm water for at least 30 minutes, then drain.

4 Preheat a grill pan and lightly brush it with oil.

5 In a medium bowl, whisk the tamarind paste with 2 tablespoons of hot (not boiling) water to soften. Add the peanut butter, coconut milk, the remaining grated ginger, remaining tamari, and crushed chillies, and whisk well.

6 Thread the marinated seitan onto the skewers and cook, turning once or twice, for 5–7 minutes or until browned on all sides. Serve immediately with the tamarind-peanut sauce.

the good stuff

Seitan is a good protein choice for vegans – it's low in fat and contains high levels of vitamin B6. A good replacement for red meat.

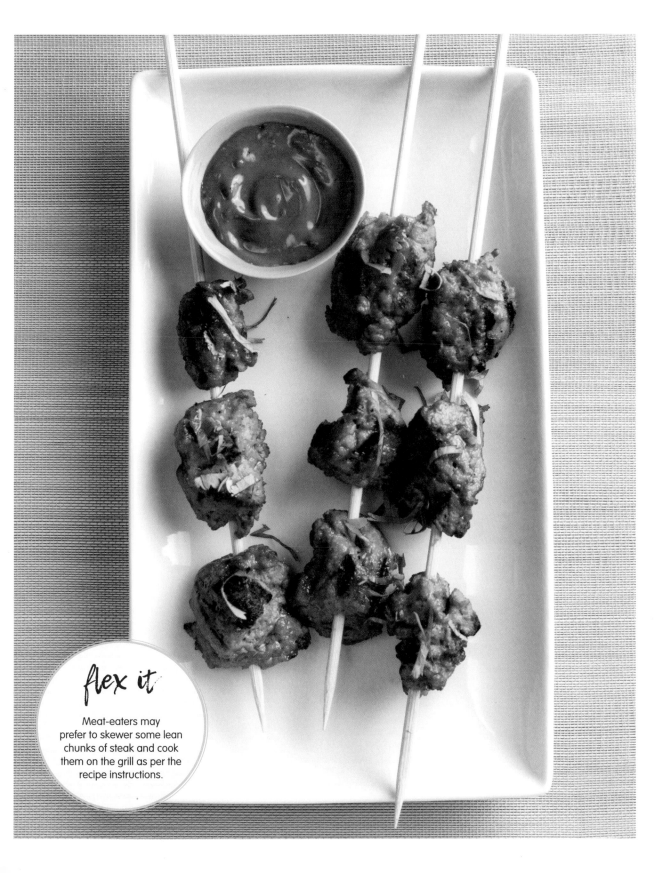

flex it

Meat-eaters may prefer to skewer some lean chunks of steak and cook them on the grill as per the recipe instructions.

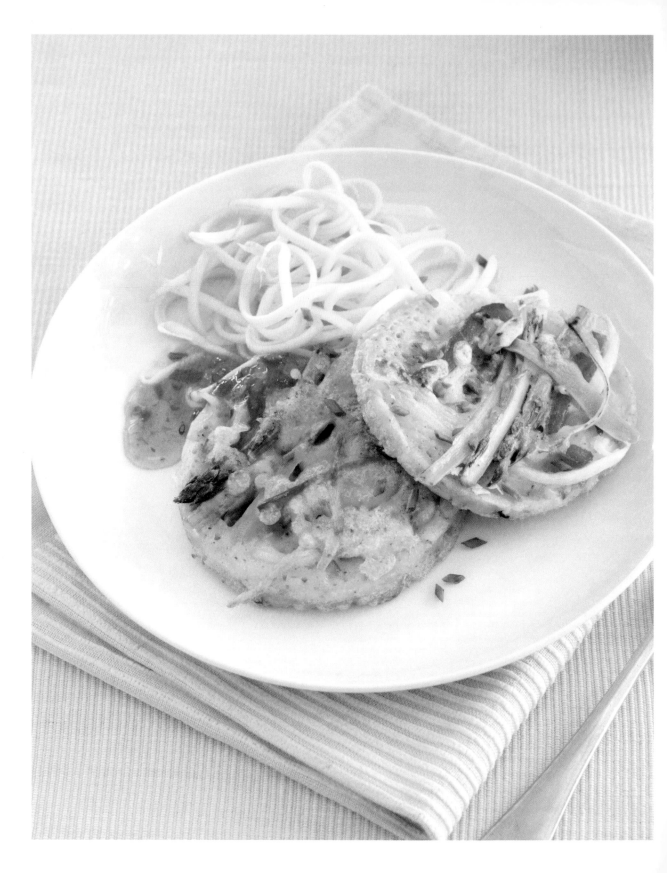

THAI-STYLE FRITTERS
with beansprouts & shredded vegetables

MAKES 8
PREP 20 MINS
COOK 25 MINS

½ **carrot**
60g (2oz) **asparagus spears**
(about 15cm/6in long)
½ small **red pepper**, deseeded
and cut into thin strips
125g (4½oz) **plain flour**
1 tsp **baking powder**
¼ tsp **ground turmeric**
¾ tsp **salt**
1 tsp grated **fresh root ginger**
1 tsp finely chopped **lemongrass**
or **lemongrass purée**
1 **garlic clove**, crushed
1 thin **red chilli**, deseeded and
finely chopped
4 **spring onions**, chopped
100g (3½oz) **beansprouts**
1 tbsp chopped **coriander**
sunflower oil, for frying
1 tbsp snipped **chives**, plus extra
to garnish
noodle and **beansprout salad**
and **sweet chilli sauce**, to serve

1 Pare the carrot into thin ribbons with a potato peeler or a mandolin. Cut the asparagus spears in half lengthways and then widthways. Set both aside with the red pepper.

2 Mix the flour with the baking powder, turmeric, salt, ginger, lemongrass, garlic, and chilli. Whisk in 250ml (8fl oz) of cold water to form a batter the consistency of thick cream. Stir in the spring onions, beansprouts, and coriander.

3 Place in 4 chef rings in a large frying pan. Add about 5mm (¼in) of sunflower oil and heat until hot, but not smoking.

4 Add about an eighth of the batter (a small ladleful) to one of the chef rings and quickly top with a few strips of each vegetable, pressing gently into the uncooked batter. Repeat with the other rings, using half the ingredients in all. Fry for 2–3 minutes until the batter is puffed up, set, and brown underneath.

5 Lift off the rings with tongs. Flip the fritters over with a fish slice and fry for a further 2 minutes to brown and cook the vegetables. Lift out with a fish slice and drain, vegetable side up, on kitchen paper. Keep warm while cooking the remaining fritters in the same way.

6 Transfer the fritters to serving plates and garnish with a few snipped chives. Serve with a noodle and beansprout salad and some sweet chilli sauce for dipping.

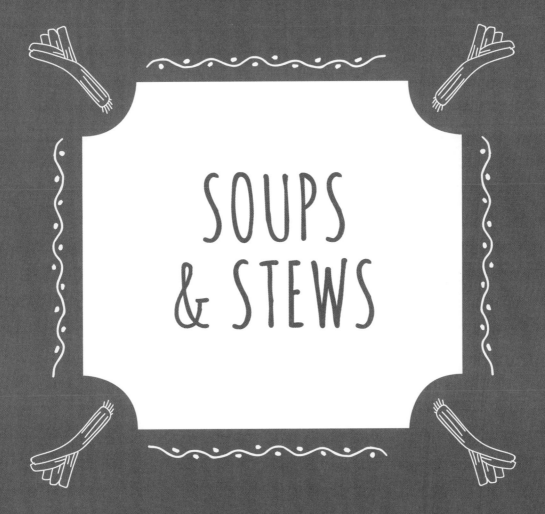

SOUPS & STEWS

CREAMY GREEN SOUP
with wheat berries, leeks, & cannellini beans

SERVES 4
PREP 15 MINS
COOK 1 HR 20 MINS, plus cooling

400g (14oz) **wheat berries**
1 tbsp **light olive oil**
1 **onion**, finely chopped
2 **garlic cloves**, crushed
4 **leeks**, trimmed and
  finely sliced
500g (1lb 2oz) **spring greens**,
  stems removed and finely sliced
750ml (1¼ pints) **vegetable stock**
2 x 400g (14oz) can **cannellini
  beans**, drained
salt and freshly ground
  black pepper

1 Put the wheat berries into a large, heavy-bottomed saucepan and cover with cold water. Bring to the boil, then reduce to a simmer and cook, uncovered, for 45–50 minutes until tender but chewy. Drain them well, and refresh under cold water, before allowing them to cool.

2 Heat the olive oil in a large saucepan over a medium heat. Add the onions and garlic and cook, stirring occasionally, for about 5 minutes.

3 Add the leeks to the pan and cook for about 10 minutes, stirring occasionally, until softened. Then add the spring greens and cook for a further 2–3 minutes, or until they wilt.

4 Pour in the vegetable stock, bring to the boil, and allow the soup to simmer for about 10 minutes. Then add the cannellini beans to the pan and stir lightly to mix. Transfer the soup to a food processor and pulse until it reaches a smooth consistency. Season to taste, if needed.

5 Return the soup to the pan and place over a medium heat for 2–3 minutes to heat through. Then stir in the wheat berries and remove from the heat. Ladle into soup bowls, season with pepper, and serve hot.

the good stuff

Wheat berries are the whole grain form of wheat. Full of fibre, low in calories and good for digestion, they make the perfect addition to a plant-based diet. Leeks perk up this dish – full of vitamins K and A, and magnesium, they keep your eyes and bones on top form.

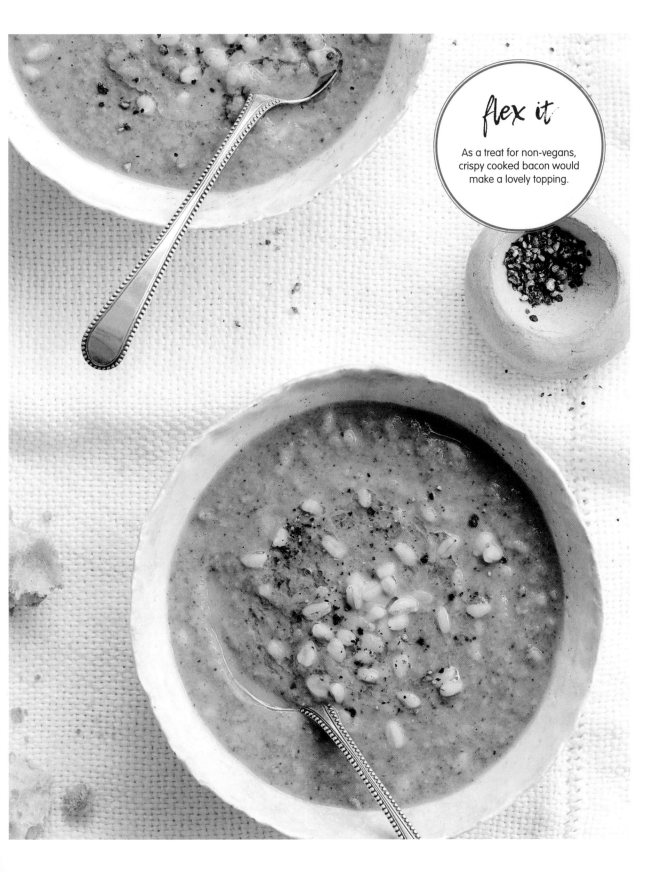

flex it

As a treat for non-vegans,
crispy cooked bacon would
make a lovely topping.

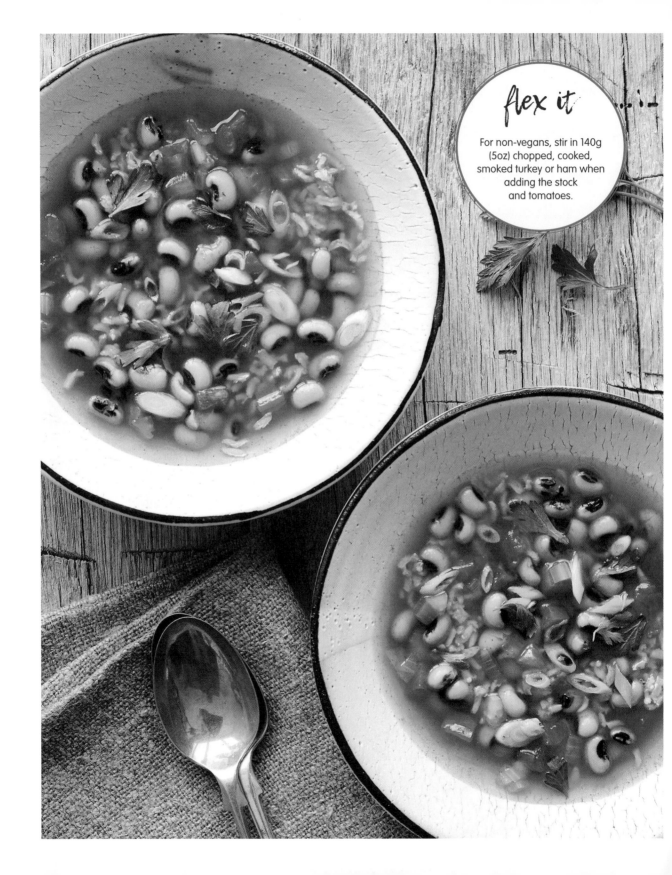

flex it

For non-vegans, stir in 140g (5oz) chopped, cooked, smoked turkey or ham when adding the stock and tomatoes.

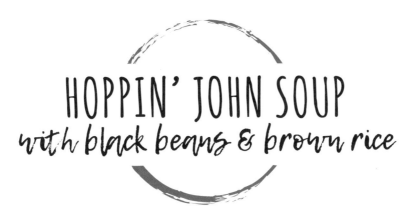

HOPPIN' JOHN SOUP
with black beans & brown rice

SERVES 6
PREP 30 MINS
COOK 40 MINS

1 tbsp **olive oil**

1 small **onion**, diced

1 small **red pepper**, deseeded
and diced

2 **celery sticks**, diced

1 **garlic clove**, finely chopped

400g (14oz) can **chopped tomatoes**

2 sprigs of **thyme**

pinch of **ground cayenne pepper**

½ tsp **smoked paprika**

1 litre (1¾ pints) **vegetable stock**

salt and freshly ground
black pepper

375g (13oz) cooked **black-eyed
beans**

175g (6oz) cooked **brown rice**

45g (1½oz) chopped
spring onion, to garnish

5g (¼oz) chopped **flat-leaf parsley**,
to garnish

1 In a large saucepan, warm the olive oil over a medium–low heat.
Add the onion and cook for 2 minutes, or until it starts to become
translucent. Add the red pepper and celery and cook for an additional
2 minutes. Add the garlic and cook for an additional minute.

2 Incorporate the tomatoes, thyme, cayenne, paprika, and stock.
Bring to the boil, then reduce the heat to low and cook, covered,
for 20 minutes. Season with salt and pepper to taste.

3 Combine the black-eyed beans and rice. Cook for 10 minutes,
or until the beans and rice are warmed through. Transfer to
serving bowls and garnish with the spring onion and parsley.

the good stuff

A combo of brown rice and black-eyed beans
contains an impressive amount of fibre and will
satisfy all your protein needs. Peppers and celery
are thrown in for plenty of vitamins A and K.

CHUNKY BUTTERNUT SQUASH SOUP
with pearl barley

SERVES 4
PREP 10 MINS
COOK 50 MINS

100g (3½oz)
  pearl barley
2 tbsp **olive oil**
1 **onion**, diced
salt and freshly ground
  black pepper
2 **carrots**, sliced into thin rounds
1 **apple**, cored and diced
1 **red pepper**, deseeded
  and diced
1 **butternut squash**, about
  900g (2lb), deseeded and
  cut into cubes
1 litre (1¾ pints) **vegetable stock**
1 tsp **ground cinnamon**
1 tsp **ground ginger**
1 tsp **sweet paprika**

1 Place the barley in a large saucepan, cover with 350ml (12fl oz) of water, and bring to the boil. Reduce the heat to medium–low and cook for 25–30 minutes, or until tender. Then remove from the heat and drain any remaining water. Set aside.

2 Meanwhile, heat the olive oil in a large Dutch oven or saucepan over a medium heat. Add the onions and season with a pinch of salt. Cook for about 8 minutes, stirring frequently, until they start to get translucent. Then add the carrots, apple, red pepper, and butternut squash. Stir to mix and pour over the vegetable stock. Cover and cook, stirring occasionally, for about 30 minutes.

3 Add the cinnamon, ginger, and paprika. Cook for a further 10 minutes. Remove from the heat and take out about 150g (5½oz) of the vegetables with a slotted spoon and set aside. Use a hand-held blender to pulse the remaining mixture until it forms a smooth purée. Add the barley and reserved vegetables, season to taste, and mix well. Serve immediately.

the good stuff

Pearl barley is a versatile cereal with more fibre than other whole grains. Chewy in texture, it offers complex carbs, and is rich in B vitamins, zinc and magnesium. Butternut squash has key antioxidants and high levels of potassium.

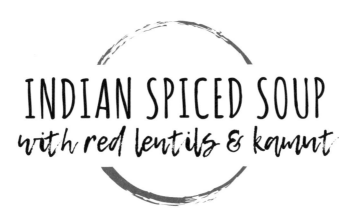

INDIAN SPICED SOUP
with red lentils & kamut

SERVES 4–6
PREP 20 MINS
COOK 40 MINS

1 tbsp **light olive oil**

1 large **onion**, finely chopped

1 **leek**, trimmed and
finely chopped

5cm (2in) piece of **fresh root
ginger**, finely chopped

2 tsp **mild curry powder**

4 **carrots**, unpeeled and
roughly chopped

300g (10oz) **red lentils**

300g (10oz) **kamut**

1.5 litres (2¾ pints) hot **vegetable
stock**, plus extra if needed

salt and freshly ground
black pepper

1 Heat the olive oil in a large saucepan over a medium heat. Add the onions and leeks and sauté for about 5 minutes. Then add the ginger and curry powder and stir to mix, adding a little water to the pan if they start to stick. Add the carrots, red lentils, and kamut to the pan and stir to mix.

2 Pour in 1 litre (1¾ pints) of the stock, reserving the rest. Cover, reduce the heat to a simmer, and cook for 30 minutes or until the lentils have broken down, the kamut is tender, and the carrots are cooked through. Check the soup occasionally and add more stock as needed.

3 Remove from the heat and use a hand-held blender to process the soup until it reaches a chunky texture, adding more stock if necessary. Taste and season with salt and pepper. Stir well to combine and serve warm.

flex it

This is a great soup for using up roast meat for a non-vegan treat. Slow-cooked lamb is really good – stir in some leftover meat just before serving.

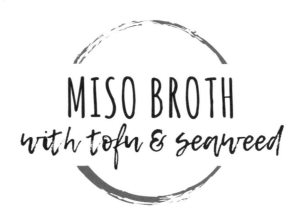

MISO BROTH
with tofu & seaweed

SERVES 1
PREP 10 MINS, plus soaking
COOK 10 MINS

2 pieces of **dried
    wakame seaweed**
10g (¼oz) **spinach** leaves
10g (¼oz) **cabbage**, shredded
1 tbsp **brown rice miso**
5cm (2in) piece of **fresh
    root ginger**, half grated, half
    finely sliced
45g (1½oz) **firm tofu**, chopped
    into cubes
sea salt and freshly ground
    black pepper
juice of 1 **lemon**
½ **spring onion**, finely sliced
½ **red chilli**, finely sliced

1 Place the wakame in a bowl and cover with hot water. Soak for 10 minutes, then drain and shred.

2 Meanwhile, steam the spinach and cabbage over boiling water for 3 minutes.

3 Pour 240ml (8fl oz) of boiling water into a saucepan, then stir in the miso paste with a fork for 2 minutes, or until it starts to dissolve. Bring to the boil, then reduce the heat to a gentle simmer and cook for 1 minute.

4 Add the grated ginger and tofu. Slowly pour in up to 120ml (4fl oz) of boiling water, tasting as you go and stopping when it tastes good to you (be careful not to dilute the miso too much). Season with salt and pepper to taste, then simmer for 5 more minutes.

5 Add the spinach, cabbage, and wakame to a serving bowl, then ladle in the miso broth and tofu. Add a squeeze of lemon juice and sprinkle with the sliced ginger, spring onion, and red chilli.

the good stuff

Miso is a paste made from fermented soya beans. It is good to have in the cupboard to whip up a healthy soup for vegans, and it also helps relieve fatigue. Dark green leafy seaweed is extremely good for you, containing high levels of calcium, and increasing iodine levels.

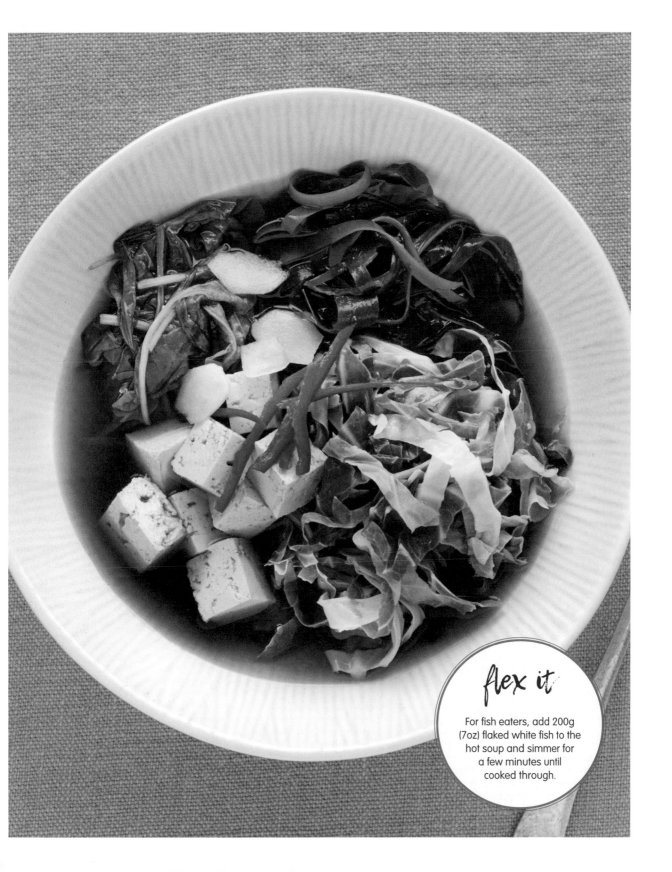

flex it

For fish eaters, add 200g
(7oz) flaked white fish to the
hot soup and simmer for
a few minutes until
cooked through.

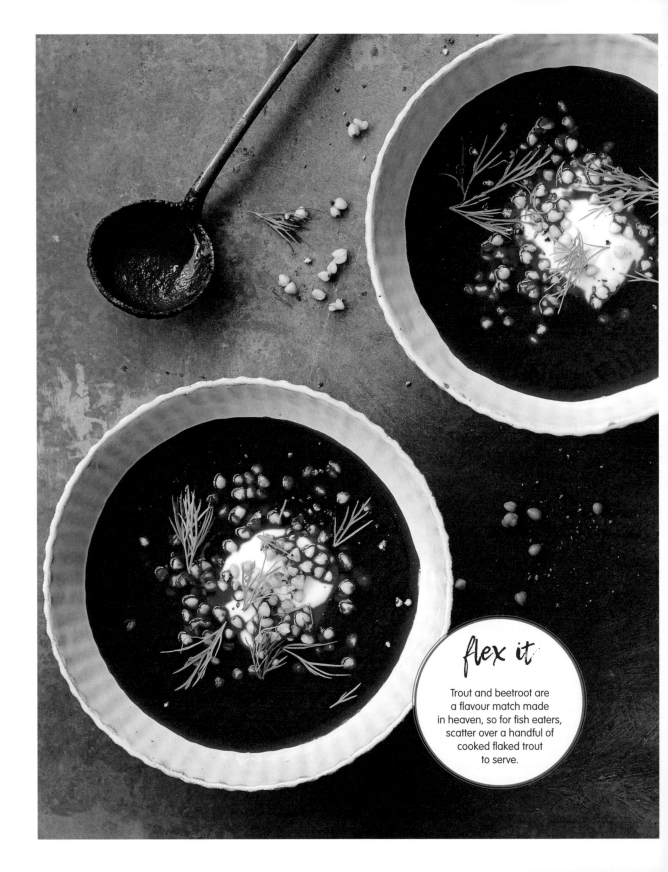

flex it

Trout and beetroot are a flavour match made in heaven, so for fish eaters, scatter over a handful of cooked flaked trout to serve.

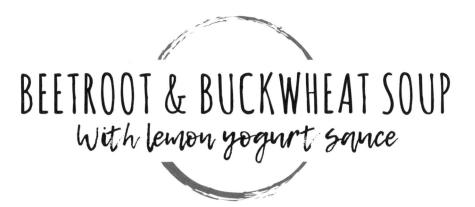

BEETROOT & BUCKWHEAT SOUP
with lemon yogurt sauce

SERVES 4
PREP 15 MINS
COOK 1 HR 5 MINS

200g (7oz) **buckwheat**
1 tbsp **light olive oil**
1 **onion**, finely chopped
750g (1lb 10oz) **beetroot**, trimmed
  and cut into small chunks
500ml (16fl oz) **vegetable stock**
400g (14oz) can **chopped tomatoes**
salt and freshly ground
  black pepper
handful of **rosemary leaves**

LEMON YOGURT SAUCE
250g (9oz) **soya yogurt** or **coconut**
  milk yogurt
juice of 1 **lemon**

1 Rinse the buckwheat, than place in a medium saucepan and cover with 500ml (16fl oz) of boiling water. Cook for about 15 minutes until tender. Set aside.

2 Heat the olive oil in a large saucepan over a medium heat. Add the onion and cook for about 5 minutes, stirring frequently, until translucent. Then add the beetroot and stock. Bring the mixture to a simmer and cook for 30–40 minutes, until the beetroot is tender.

3 Add the tomatoes to the pan and cook for 2–3 minutes. Transfer the soup to a food processor and pulse until it reaches a smooth consistency. Season to taste, if needed. Pour the soup back into the pan and heat through over a low heat for 2–3 minutes. Remove from the heat.

4 For the sauce, place the ingredients in a bowl and mix to combine. Divide the soup between 4 bowls and top with the sauce. Then add equal quantities of the buckwheat, garnish with rosemary, and serve hot.

the good stuff

Reap the health benefits of adding beetroot to your plant-based diet – it is packed with iron, which reduces the risk of anemia. Beetroot also contains silica, an important component needed for the body to use calcium efficiently. Its natural sweetness is good for sating sugar cravings.

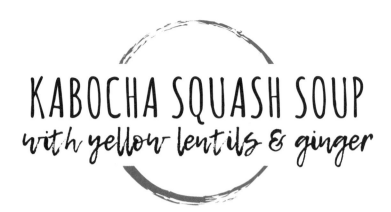

KABOCHA SQUASH SOUP
with yellow lentils & ginger

SERVES 4
PREP 20 MINS
COOK 1 HR 40 MINS

1 **kabocha squash** or **butternut squash**, deseeded and cut into quarters
2 tbsp **olive oil**
1 **carrot**, chopped
1 **onion**, chopped
1 **celery stick**, chopped
1.25 litres (2 pints) **vegetable stock**
325g (11oz) **yellow lentils**
2 tsp **curry powder**
½ tsp **ground ginger**
165ml (5.6fl oz) can **unsweetened coconut milk**
salt and freshly ground **black pepper**
1 **lime**, cut into 4 wedges
unsweetened, toasted coconut flakes, to garnish

1 Preheat the oven to 180°C (350°F/Gas 4). Place the squash quarters cut-side up on a baking tray and drizzle with 1 tablespoon of olive oil. Roast for 40 minutes, or until tender. Leave to cool.

2 Meanwhile, in a large saucepan, heat the remaining 1 tablespoon of oil over a medium heat. Add the carrot, onion, and celery and cook for 3 minutes, or until translucent. Add 750ml (1¼ pints) of stock and the yellow lentils and bring to the boil. Reduce to a simmer and cook, covered, for 45 minutes to 1 hour, until the lentils are tender. To ensure there is enough liquid for the lentils to absorb, add up to 500ml (15fl oz) of additional stock as needed.

3 When the lentils are tender, scoop the roasted squash from its skin and add the flesh to the pan. Stir in the curry powder and ginger and heat through. With a blender or hand-held blender, purée until smooth. Stir in the coconut milk and heat thoroughly. Season with salt and pepper to taste. Serve with a lime wedge and some coconut flakes for scattering over.

the good stuff

Yellow lentils are a nutritional powerhouse; they are full of protein and an excellent source of folate, the all-important B12 which must be included in a vegan diet.

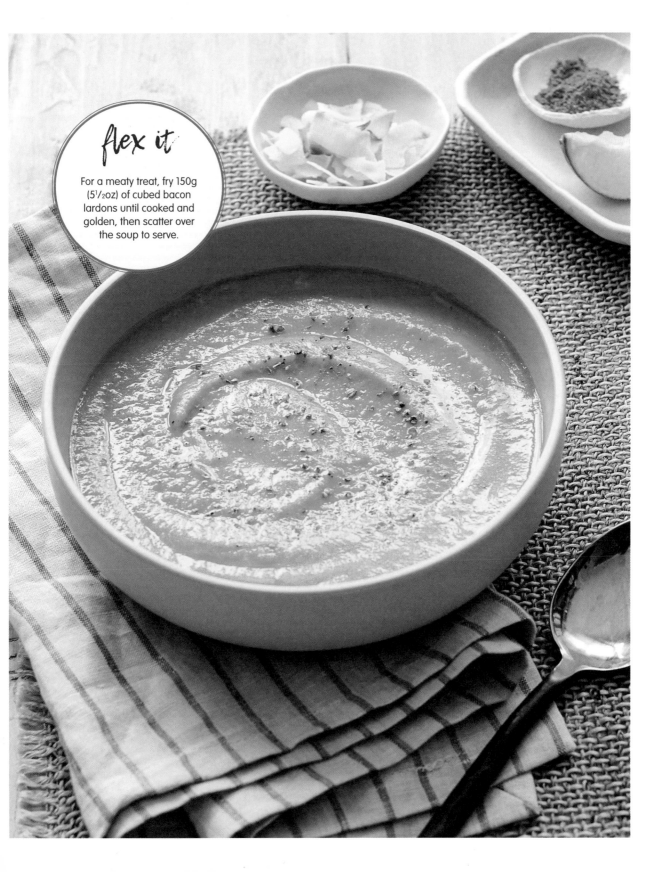

flex it

For a meaty treat, fry 150g
(5½oz) of cubed bacon
lardons until cooked and
golden, then scatter over
the soup to serve.

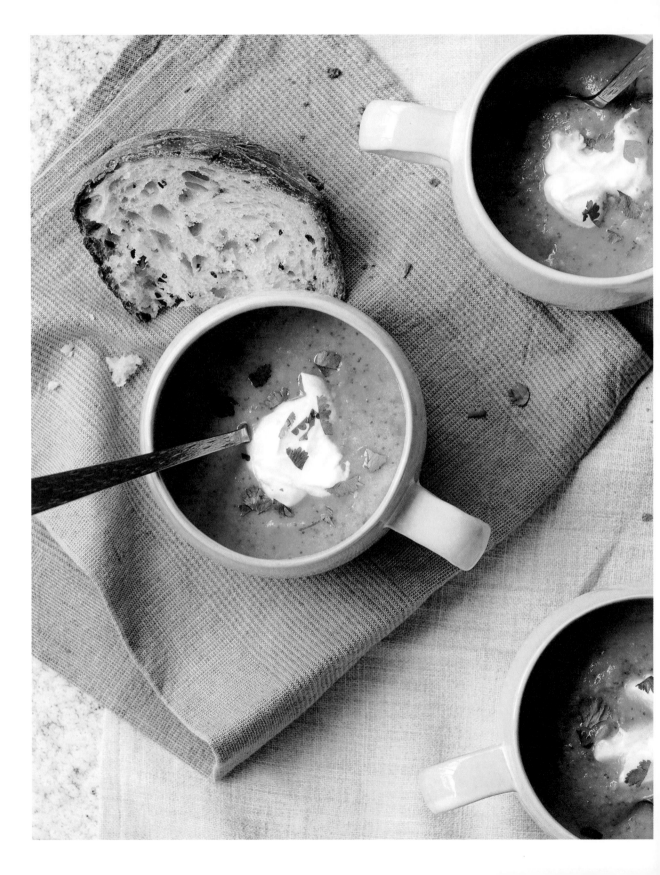

SWEET POTATO, TEFF, & PEANUT SOUP
topped with coconut milk yogurt

SERVES 6–8
PREP 15 MINS
COOK 45 MINS

100g (3½oz) **teff**

1 tbsp **light olive oil**

1 **onion**, finely chopped

2 **garlic cloves**, finely chopped

1 tbsp **ground cumin**

400g (14oz) can **chopped tomatoes**

700g (1lb 8oz) **sweet potatoes**,
   unpeeled and cut into cubes

1 litre (1¾ pints) **vegetable stock**

100g (3½oz) **smooth peanut butter**

salt and freshly ground
   black pepper

200g (7oz) **coconut milk yogurt**,
   to serve

6 tbsp roughly chopped **coriander
   leaves**, to garnish

1 Place 400ml (14fl oz) of water in a large saucepan and bring to the boil. Add the teff and reduce the heat to a simmer. Cook for 10 minutes, stirring constantly, until all the water has been absorbed. Remove from the heat and set aside.

2 Meanwhile, heat the olive oil in a large saucepan over a medium heat. Add the onions and garlic and sauté for about 5 minutes or until the onions have softened. Then add the cumin and sauté for a further 2 minutes.

3 Add the tomatoes, sweet potatoes, and stock to the pan and reduce the heat to a simmer. Cover and cook for 30 minutes or until the potatoes are soft. Remove from the heat and use a hand-held blender to process the soup until smooth. Then add the peanut butter and process until fully incorporated.

4 Add the teff to the soup and stir through. Return the pan to a medium heat and warm through for 2–3 minutes. Remove from the heat and season to taste, if needed. Ladle into soup bowls and top with a spoonful of yogurt. Sprinkle over the coriander and serve hot.

the good stuff

Teff is a really good grain to include in a plant-based diet. It has high levels of vitamins and minerals and five times the iron found in wheat. This iron is also easily absorbed because teff contains low levels of phytic acid.

SUMMER PEA, MINT, & AVOCADO SOUP
with quinoa

SERVES 4
PREP 10 MINS
COOK 25 MINS

50g (1¾oz) **quinoa**
2 **avocados**
500g (1lb 2oz) **frozen peas**
20g (¾oz) chopped **mint**, plus extra
  to garnish
1 litre (1¾ pints) **unsweetened
  almond milk**

1 Rinse the quinoa under running water, drain, and place in a lidded saucepan. Cover with 250ml (9fl oz) of water and bring to the boil.

2 Reduce the heat to a simmer, cover, and cook for 15–20 minutes, or until almost all the liquid has been absorbed and the quinoa is fluffy. Remove from the heat, drain any remaining water, and set aside to cool.

3 Scoop out the flesh from the avocados and place in a food processor. Add the peas, mint, and half the milk, and pulse until smooth. Then add the remaining milk and pulse until fully blended.

4 Divide the soup equally between 4 soup bowls. Top with equal quantities of the cooled quinoa. Garnish with some mint and serve immediately.

the good stuff

Peas offer a super serving of vitamin K. With relatively high levels of protein, they also fill you up and satisfy, so you're not left feeling hungry.

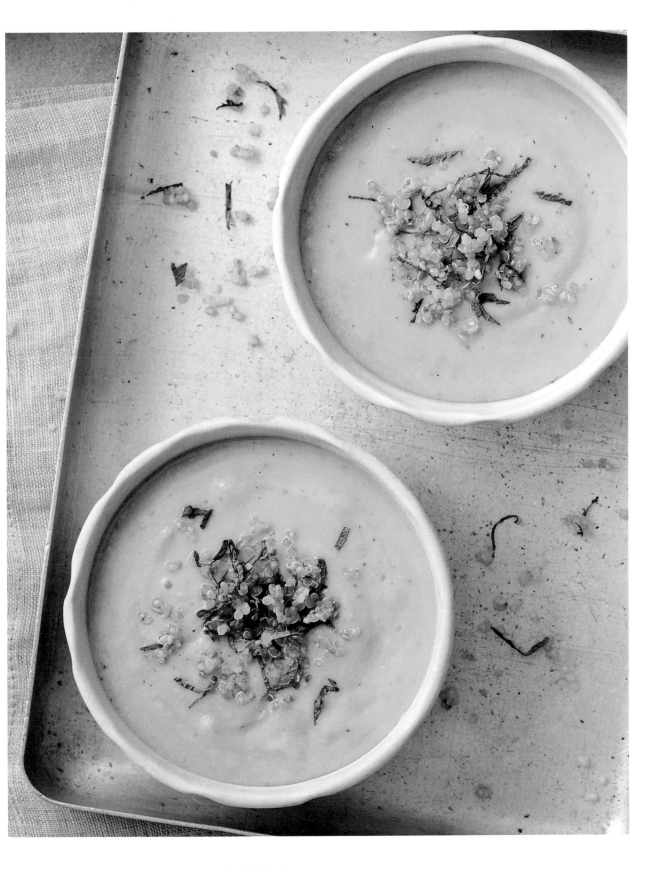

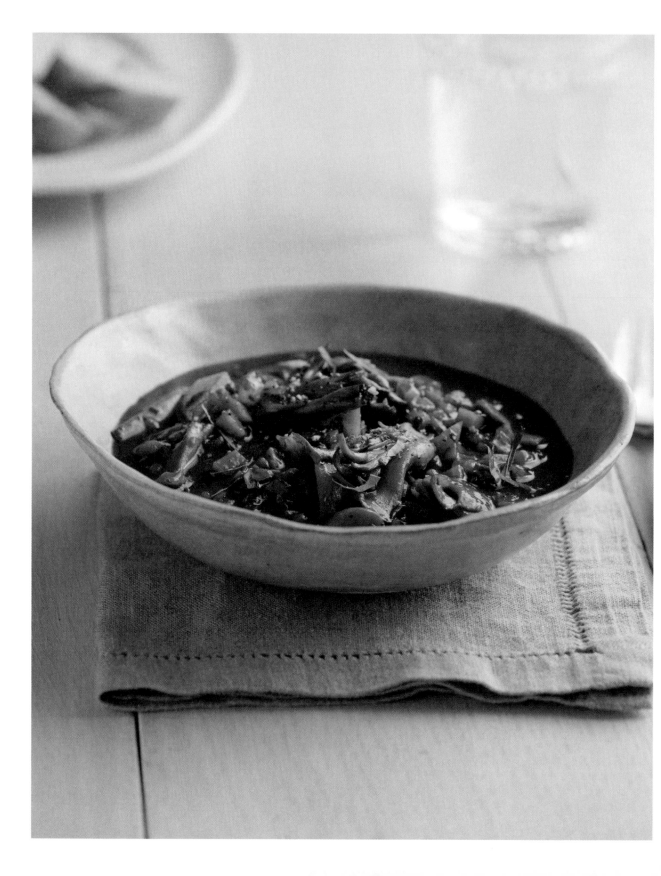

MEATY MUSHROOM STEW
with red wine & balsamic vinegar

SERVES 6
PREP 15 MINS
COOK 30 MINS

4 tbsp **extra virgin olive oil**

2 **onions**, finely chopped

1 small **shallot**, halved and
  finely chopped

2 **celery sticks**, finely chopped

1 large **carrot**, finely chopped

300g (10oz) tiny white **button
  mushrooms**, halved

225g (8oz) **hen of the woods
  mushrooms**, sliced

225g (8oz) **chanterelle
  mushrooms**, sliced

3 **garlic cloves**, finely chopped

1 tsp **sea salt**, plus extra to taste

½ tsp freshly ground **black pepper**,
  plus more to taste

1 tbsp **sweet Hungarian paprika**

1 tsp **dried thyme**

1 tsp **dried dill**

2 tbsp **plain flour**

720–960ml (1 pint 4fl oz–1¾ pints)
  vegetable or **mushroom stock**

240ml (8fl oz) **dry red wine**

1 large **Desiree potato**, peeled
  and diced

4 tbsp finely chopped **flat-leaf
  parsley**

1 tbsp **balsamic vinegar**

1 Heat 2 tablespoons of olive oil in a 4-litre (7-pint) large, deep-sided pan over a medium–high heat. Add the onions and shallot, and cook, stirring frequently, for 5 minutes.

2 Add the celery, carrot, the mushrooms, and garlic, and cook, stirring frequently, for about 10 minutes or until the mushrooms begin to turn golden. Add the remaining olive oil as the mushrooms start to stick to the pan.

3 Stir in the salt, black pepper, sweet Hungarian paprika, thyme, and dill. Add the flour to the mushroom mixture and stir for 2 minutes.

4 Add 720ml (1 pint 4fl oz) of vegetable or mushroom stock, the red wine, and potato, and bring to the boil. Reduce the heat to medium and cook, stirring often, for 10 minutes or until the stew is thickened and vegetables are tender. Add additional stock if the stew is too thick for your liking.

5 Remove from the heat, and stir in the flat-leaf parsley and balsamic vinegar. Taste, add more salt and black pepper if needed, and serve. The stew will keep in the fridge for up to 5 days and is even more delicious the next day.

the good stuff

Mushrooms contain healing benefits, including antimicrobial and antibacterial properties. They are also packed with vitamins C and D, potassium, and several beneficial minerals that may be harder to get in a plant-based diet, such as selenium, copper, iron, phosphorus, and potassium.

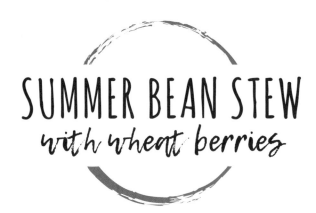

SUMMER BEAN STEW
with wheat berries

SERVES 4
PREP 20 MINS, plus soaking
COOK 55 MINS

100g (3½oz) **wheat berries**
1 tbsp **light olive oil**
1 **onion**, finely chopped
2 **garlic cloves**,
    finely chopped
2 **celery sticks**,
    finely chopped
2 **yellow** or **red peppers**,
    deseeded and diced
1 **courgette**, diced
500ml (16fl oz) **vegetable stock**
400g (14oz) can **haricot beans**,
    drained
400g (14oz) can **borlotti beans**,
    drained
400g (14oz) can **chopped
    tomatoes**
2 tsp **Italian herb seasoning**
salt and freshly ground
    black pepper
handful of **basil leaves**,
    to garnish

1 Place the wheat berries in a large bowl and cover with water. Leave to soak overnight or for at least 8 hours. Then drain any remaining water and rinse under running water. Drain well and set aside.

2 Heat the oil in a large soup pot over a medium heat. Add the onions and garlic and sauté for about 3 minutes or until the onions are translucent. Add the celery and sauté for a further 2 minutes. Then add the peppers and courgette and cook for 3 minutes, stirring frequently.

3 Add the stock, wheat berries, both lots of beans, tomatoes, and Italian seasoning. Stir well and reduce the heat to a simmer. Cover and cook for 45 minutes, until the vegetables and wheat berries are tender. Season to taste, if needed, and remove from the heat. Serve hot, garnished with basil.

the good stuff

This bowl of stew will provide you with your daily quota of fibre, thanks to the multitasking beans, which are also 1 of your 5-a-day.

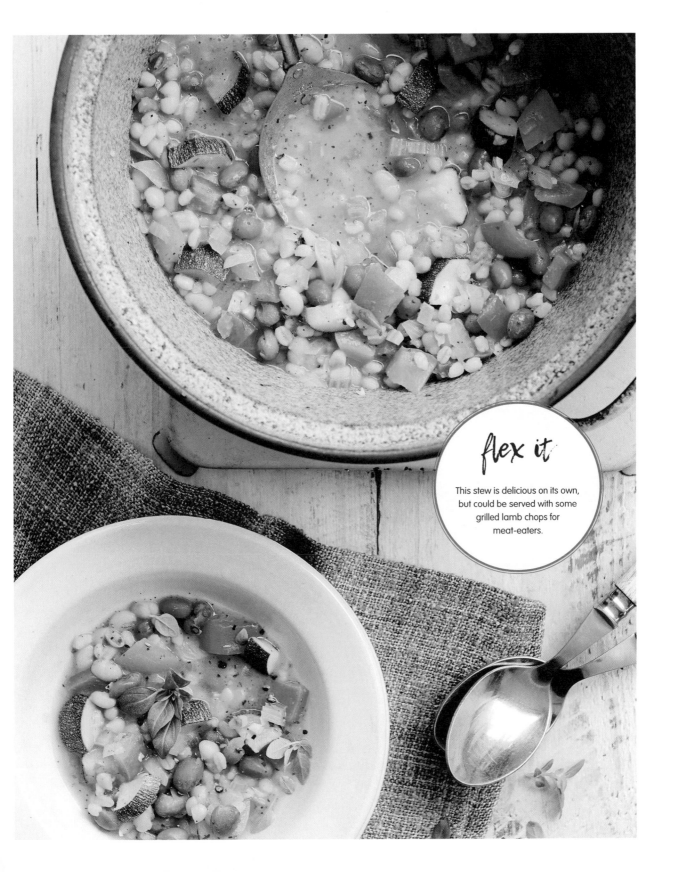

flex it

This stew is delicious on its own, but could be served with some grilled lamb chops for meat-eaters.

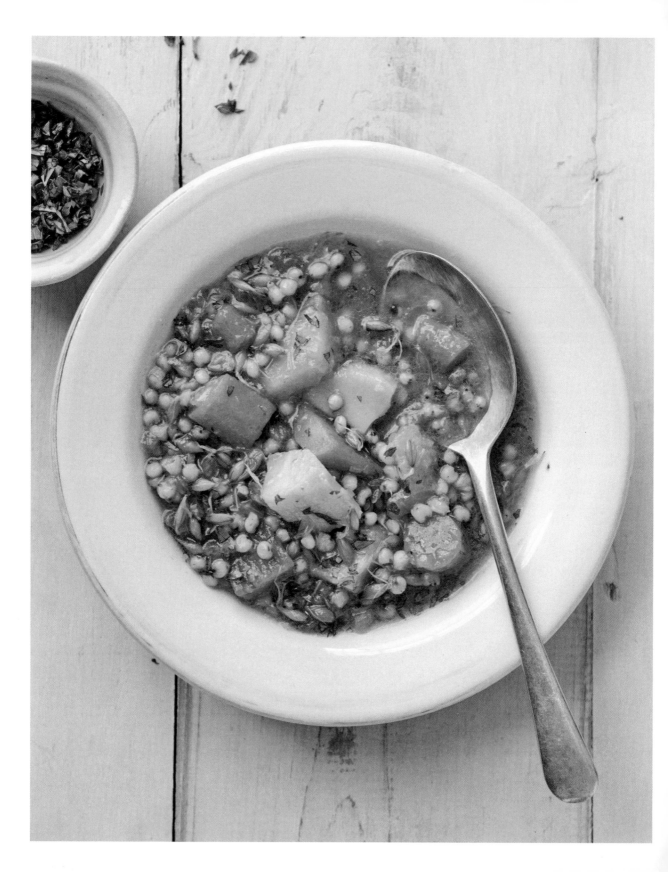

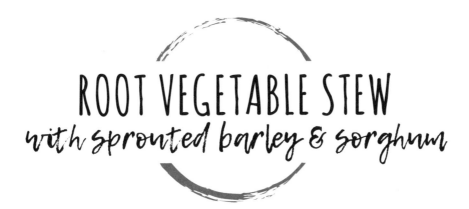

ROOT VEGETABLE STEW
with sprouted barley & sorghum

SERVES 4
PREP 10 MINS
COOK 1 HR 10 MINS

4 tbsp **olive oil**
300g (10oz) **young turnips**, chopped
300g (10oz) **carrots**, chopped
300g (10oz) **parsnips**, chopped
1 **onion**, finely chopped
2 **celery sticks**, peeled, and finely chopped
100g (3½oz) **sprouted barley**
200g (7oz) **sorghum grains**
2 litres (3½ pints) **vegetable stock**
1 tsp chopped **thyme leaves**
salt and freshly ground **black pepper**
10g (¼oz) finely chopped **flat-leaf parsley**

1 In a casserole dish or large, heavy-based saucepan with a lid, heat the olive oil over a medium heat. Add the turnips, carrots, and parsnips and cook for 5 minutes, turning occasionally, until they begin to brown. Remove them from the pan and set aside.

2 Add the onion and celery to the pan and cook over a medium heat for 3 minutes until they start to soften, but do not brown. Add the barley and sorghum and cook for another 2 minutes until the grains start to colour.

3 Add the vegetable stock and thyme, and season well with salt and pepper. Bring to the boil, then reduce the heat to a simmer, cover, and cook for 40 minutes; the grains will be part-cooked.

4 Remove the lid and increase the heat. Add the browned root vegetables and parsley and return to the boil. Reduce the heat to a simmer and cook, uncovered, for a final 20 minutes until the vegetables have softened and the stock has reduced. Season with salt and pepper, if needed, and serve immediately.

the good stuff

As well as its robust flavour, barley is a good source of micronutrients – sprouted grains activate enzymes, improve amino acids, have a high vitamin content, and are easier to digest.

POSOLE (MEXICAN VEGETABLE STEW)
mushrooms & hominy

SERVES 4–6
PREP 10 MINS
COOK 20 MINS

3 tbsp **olive oil**
1 large **onion**, finely chopped
2 **carrots**, cut into 5mm
 (½in) rounds
225g (8oz) **chestnut mushrooms**,
 thinly sliced
2 **garlic cloves**, finely chopped
3 tbsp **dried ground New Mexico
 chilli powder**
1 tsp **ground cumin**
1 tsp **sea salt**
½ tsp **dried oregano**
960ml (1¾ pints) **vegetable stock**
425g (15oz) **hominy** or **sweetcorn**,
 rinsed and drained
1 **courgette**, trimmed, quartered
 lengthways, and cut into 1cm
 (½in) chunks
juice of 1 **lime**
2 tbsp finely chopped
 coriander leaves

1 Heat the olive oil in a large, deep-sided pan or stockpot over a medium–high heat. Add the onion and cook, stirring frequently and adjusting the heat as necessary, for 5 minutes.

2 Stir in the carrots and mushrooms, and cook for 5 minutes.

3 Add the garlic and stir for 1 minute.

4 Sprinkle the chilli powder, cumin, salt, and oregano over the vegetable mixture and stir for 30 seconds.

5 Add the vegetable stock, bring to a simmer, and cook for 5 minutes.

6 Add the hominy or sweetcorn and courgette, bring to the boil, reduce the heat to medium–low, and cook for 10 minutes.

7 Remove from the heat, stir in the lime juice and coriander and serve.

the good stuff

Get 3 of your 5-a-day in this tasty pot. Carrots are a low-calorie food stacked with vitamin A, which is needed to keep your vision at its best.

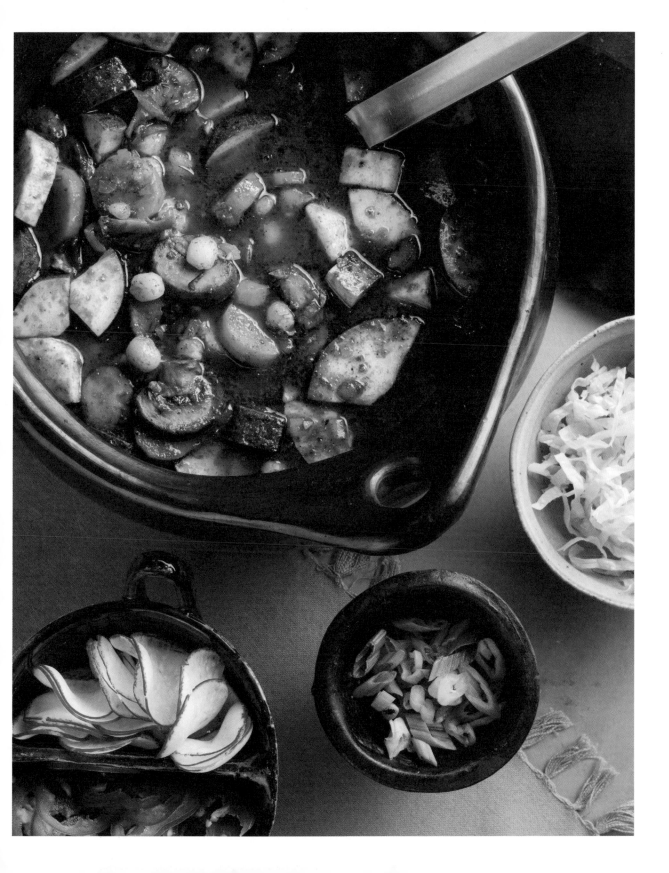

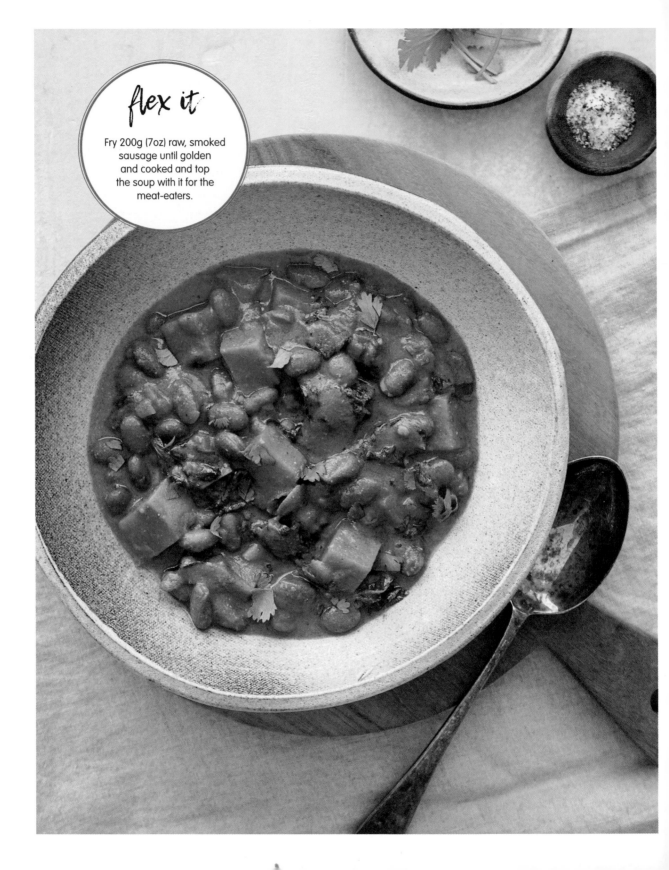

flex it

Fry 200g (7oz) raw, smoked sausage until golden and cooked and top the soup with it for the meat-eaters.

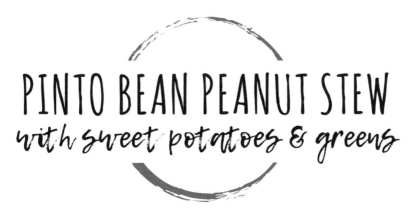

PINTO BEAN PEANUT STEW
with sweet potatoes & greens

SERVES 6
PREP 25 MINS
COOK 45 MINS

1 tbsp **coconut oil**
1 small **onion**, chopped
1 **garlic clove**, finely chopped
1 large **sweet potato**, peeled and
   cut into 3cm (1in) cubes
1 tsp **ancho chilli powder**
½ tsp **cayenne pepper**
400g (14oz) **chopped tomatoes**
600ml (1 pint) **vegetable stock**
125g (4½oz) **smooth peanut butter**
450g (1lb) cooked **pinto beans**
45g (1½oz) chopped **leafy greens**
salt and freshly ground
   black pepper
chopped **coriander leaves**,
   to garnish

1 In a medium stockpot, heat the coconut oil over a medium–low heat until shimmering. Add the onion and cook for 2–3 minutes until soft. Add the garlic and cook for 1 minute.

2 Add the sweet potato, ancho chilli powder, and cayenne. Stir to combine. Pour in the chopped tomatoes and stock. Bring to the boil then reduce to a simmer and cook, uncovered, for 5 minutes.

3 Stir in the peanut butter. Return to the boil then reduce the heat and simmer, covered, for 10 minutes.

4 Fold in the pinto beans and greens. Return to the boil once more, then reduce to a simmer and cook, covered, for 15 minutes, or until the greens are tender. Season with salt and pepper to taste. Garnish with the coriander and serve immediately.

the good stuff

Canned tomatoes, full of carotenoids, are a wonder staple for the store cupboard. There are also plenty of dark leafy greens in this, which are rich in minerals, particularly iron.

BURGERS, SANDWICHES, & WRAPS

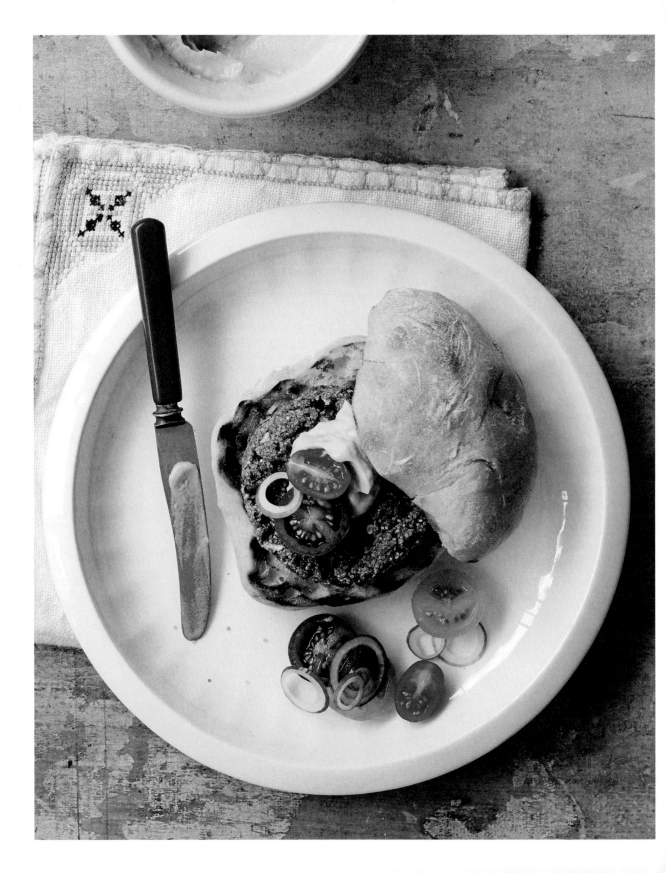

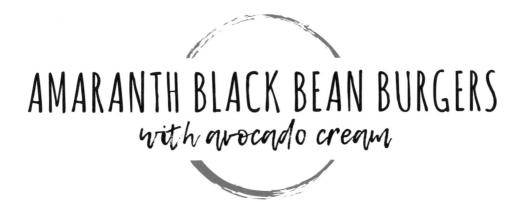

AMARANTH BLACK BEAN BURGERS
with avocado cream

MAKES 6
PREP 15 MINS, plus cooling
COOK 45 MINS

60g (2oz) **amaranth**
400g (14oz) can **black beans**,
  drained
1 small **red onion**, finely chopped
½ tsp **garlic granules**
  or ¼ tsp **garlic powder**
½ tsp **chilli flakes**
10g (¼oz) **rolled oats**
¼ tsp **salt**
6 **burger buns**, to serve
handful of **cherry tomatoes**,
  thinly sliced, to serve
1 small **red onion**, sliced
  into rings, to serve

AVOCADO CREAM
2 **avocados**
juice of 1 **lemon**
pinch of **salt**

1 Place the amaranth in a large saucepan and cover with 130ml (4¼fl oz) of water. Bring to the boil, then reduce to a simmer, and cook for 12 minutes or until all the water has been absorbed. Remove from the heat, drain any remaining water, and leave to cool slightly.

2 Preheat the oven to 200°C (400°F/Gas 6). Grease and line a baking tray with baking parchment. Transfer the amaranth to a large bowl. Add the beans, onions, garlic, and chilli flakes. Mix well, using the back of a fork to mash the ingredients together. Then add the rolled oats and salt to the mixture. Mix until well incorporated.

3 Divide the mixture into 6 equal portions and shape into balls. Gently press down each ball to form a burger patty about 7.5cm (3in) in diameter. Place the burgers on the prepared baking tray and transfer to the oven. Bake for 30 minutes or until they are firm to the touch and crispy on the outside.

4 For the avocado cream, scoop out the flesh from the avocado and place in a food processor. Add the lemon juice and salt and pulse until smooth. Place the burgers in the buns and top with the avocado cream. Serve with the tomatoes and onions.

the good stuff

Amaranth contains plenty of protein and all the amino acids your body needs. It is also a good source of calcium and has high levels of zinc.

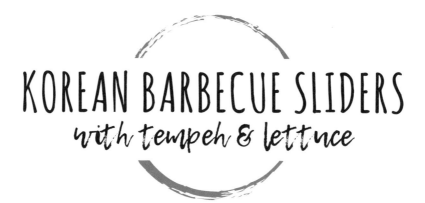

KOREAN BARBECUE SLIDERS
with tempeh & lettuce

MAKES 8
PREP 15 MINS, plus marinating
COOK 20 MINS

225g (8oz) **tempeh**
125ml (4fl oz) **low-sodium tamari**
55g (scant 2oz) **brown sugar**
3 **garlic cloves**, finely chopped
1 tbsp **sambal oelek**
1 tbsp finely chopped **fresh root ginger**
1 tbsp plus 2 tsp **rice vinegar**
2 tsp **toasted sesame oil**
1 tbsp **cornflour**
1 tsp **toasted sesame seeds**
1 tsp **granulated sugar**
8 **small buns**, such as **wholemeal rolls** or **slider buns**
50g (1¾oz) **romaine lettuce**, shredded
60g (2oz) **radishes**, thinly sliced

1 Place the tempeh in a small frying pan, cover with water, set over a medium heat, and bring to a simmer. Cover and cook for 10 minutes. Remove the lid, drain, and cool. Cut into 2 horizontal slices, then cut each into 4 equal pieces, so you have 8 small "burgers". Place the tempeh slices in a shallow pan that will accommodate them in a single layer.

2 In a small pan over a high heat, combine 120ml (4fl oz) of the tamari, brown sugar, garlic, sambal oelek, ginger, 1 tablespoon of the rice vinegar, and 1 teaspoon of the sesame oil. Bring to the boil.

3 In a small bowl, combine the cornflour and 1 tablespoon of water until smooth. Add to the sauce and cook for 1 minute or until thickened.

4 Pour the hot barbecue sauce over the tempeh, and marinate at room temperature for 30 minutes (or up to 24 hours in the fridge).

5 Preheat a grill to high. In a bowl, whisk together the 2 teaspoons of rice vinegar, remaining 1 teaspoon of tamari, remaining 1 teaspoon of sesame oil, toasted sesame seeds, and granulated sugar. Set aside.

6 Grill the tempeh slices, turning once, until they're hot and crispy. Place 1 tempeh slice on each bun.

7 In a small bowl, toss the romaine lettuce and radishes with the dressing. Distribute among the buns and serve immediately.

the good stuff

Tempeh is high in protein and also rich in minerals, copper, and manganese – which helps to clear glutamate, a nerve toxin, from your brain.

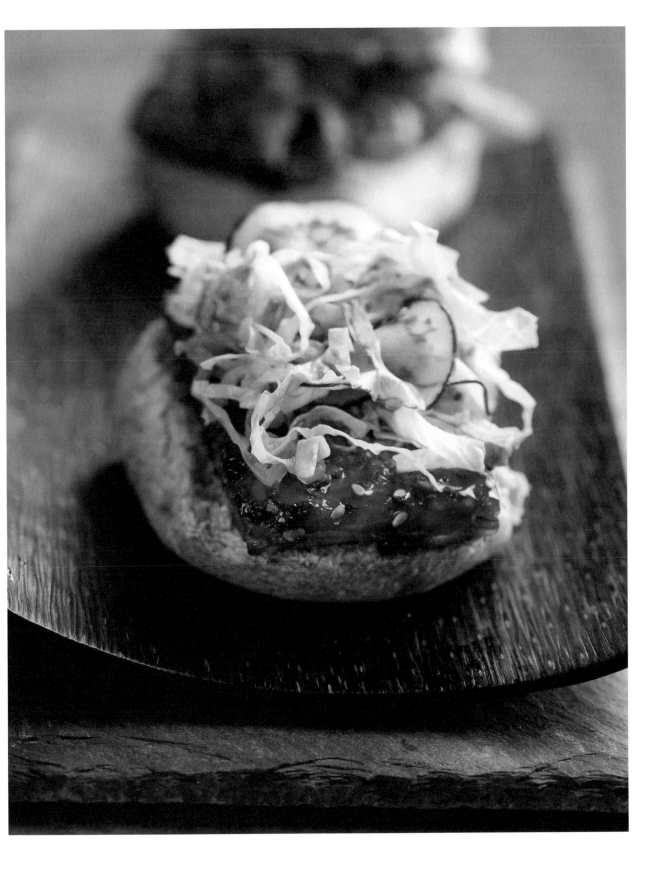

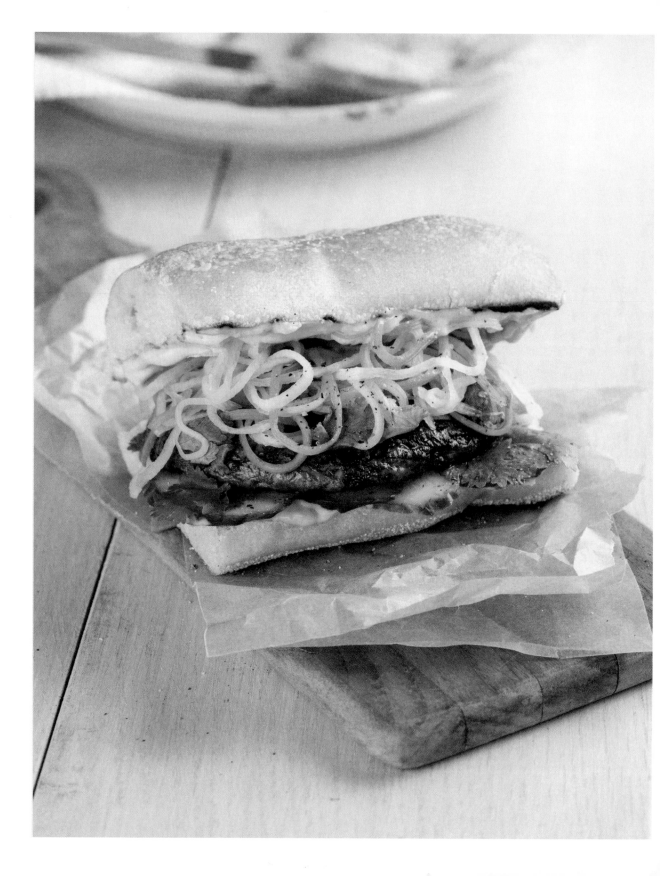

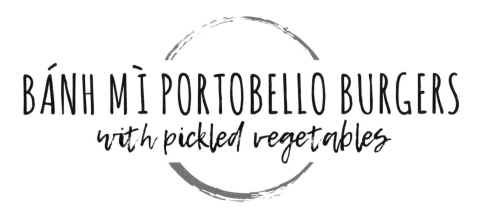

BÁNH MÌ PORTOBELLO BURGERS
with pickled vegetables

SERVES 4
PREP 40 MINS
COOK 10 MINS

4 large **portobello mushrooms**,
  stems removed
2 tbsp **plant-based mayonnaise**
1 tsp **Sriracha hot sauce**
4 x 10cm (4in) pieces crusty
  baguette, split
½ **cucumber**, thinly sliced
coriander leaves (optional)

MARINADE
juice of 1 **lime**
2 tbsp **low-sodium tamari**
  or **soy sauce**
1 tsp **toasted sesame oil**
½ tsp **garlic powder**
½ tsp **ground ginger**

PICKLED VEGETABLES
1 small **daikon radish**, peeled
  and shredded
1 **carrot**, shredded
4 tbsp **rice vinegar**
1 tbsp **sugar**
1 tsp **sea salt**

1 In a small bowl, whisk together the marinade ingredients. Wipe each mushroom clean with damp kitchen paper, place the mushrooms in a zip-lock plastic bag, pour in the marinade, seal the bag, and shake gently to distribute the marinade. Set aside.

2 To make the pickled vegetables, gently toss the daikon radish and carrot in a medium bowl. In a small saucepan over a medium heat, combine the rice vinegar, sugar, and salt with 4 tablespoons of water. Bring to the boil, stirring to dissolve the sugar and salt. Pour the vinegar mixture over the daikon and carrot, stir. Set aside for about 30 minutes, then drain.

3 In another small bowl, whisk together the plant-based mayonnaise and the Sriracha hot sauce.

4 Preheat a grill to high or set a grill pan over a high heat on your hob. Place the mushrooms on the grill, gill side down, and cook for 3 minutes. Turn them over and cook for a further 2 minutes or until the mushrooms are juicy and tender. During the last minute of mushroom cooking time, place the baguette pieces on the grill, split side down, to toast.

5 To assemble the sandwiches, spread one-quarter of the mayonnaise mixture on one side of each baguette and add a layer of cucumber slices. Place 1 mushroom burger on each sandwich and top with one-quarter of the drained pickled vegetables. Garnish with coriander leaves (if using), and serve immediately.

PUY LENTIL & MUSHROOM BURGERS
with lettuce, tomato, & onion

MAKES 4
PREP 15 MINS, plus chilling
COOK 40–45 MINS

100g (3½oz) **Puy lentils**
3 tbsp **olive oil**, plus extra
   for frying the burgers
1 **onion**, finely chopped
450g (1lb) **portobello mushrooms**,
   wiped, trimmed, and
   roughly chopped
2 **garlic cloves**, crushed
1 tsp **thyme leaves**, chopped
1 tbsp finely chopped
   flat-leaf parsley
1 tbsp **balsamic vinegar**
60g (2oz) **fresh white breadcrumbs**
1 tbsp **nutritional yeast**
salt and freshly ground
   black pepper
wholemeal buns, **lettuce leaves**,
   tomato, and **red onion** slices,
   to serve

1 Place the lentils in a saucepan of cold water and bring to the boil. Reduce to a low simmer, skimming off any foam from the top, and cook for 15 minutes until just soft. Drain and rinse, then leave to cool.

2 Heat 1 tablespoon of the olive oil in a large, non-stick frying pan. Cook the onion over a medium heat for 5 minutes, until softened but not brown. Add the remaining oil and the chopped mushrooms, and cook for a further 15–20 minutes, until they break down and there is no moisture left in the pan. Add the garlic, thyme, and parsley and cook for a further minute, until the garlic is fragrant. Add the balsamic vinegar and remove from the heat.

3 Put the mushroom mixture, cooled lentils, breadcrumbs, and nutritional yeast into a food processor and season well. Pulse carefully until it is just mixed and still has some texture.

4 Allow the mixture to cool for 5 minutes. Shape the cooled mixture into 4 equal-sized patties and chill, covered, for 30 minutes to allow them to firm up.

5 Clean the frying pan with a piece of kitchen paper. Heat a little oil in the pan and cook the burgers over a medium heat for 3–4 minutes on each side, until well browned and cooked through. Serve in wholemeal buns, with your choice of accompaniments.

the good stuff

Protein-packed Puy lentils are rich in soluble fibre, which stabilises your blood sugar and makes you feel full for longer. Onions are surprisingly high in vitamin C and full of probiotic fibre.

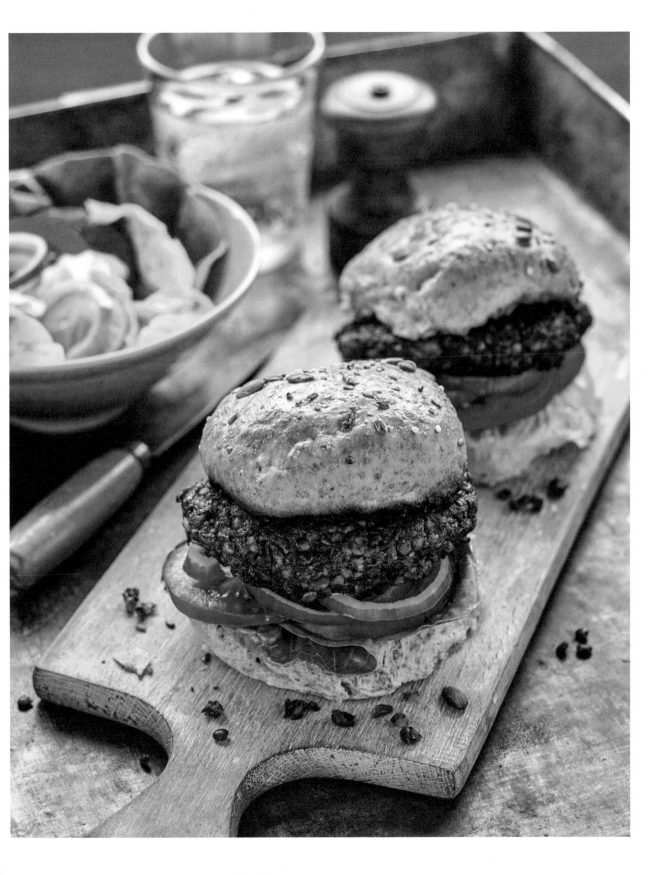

FALAFEL BURGERS
with tahini & garlic dressing

SERVES 4
PREP 15 MINS
COOK 10 MINS

1 tbsp **ground flax seeds**

4 tbsp **extra virgin olive oil**

1 **onion**, finely chopped

2 tsp **ground cumin**

1 tsp **ground coriander**

½ tsp **sea salt**

½ tsp freshly ground **black pepper**

1 tsp **lemon** zest

juice of 2 **lemons**

4 tbsp finely chopped **coriander
    leaves**

2 tbsp finely chopped **flat-leaf
    parsley**

2 x 400g (14oz) can **chickpeas**,
    drained and rinsed, 4 tbsp
    liquid reserved

60g (2oz) **fresh breadcrumbs**

3 tbsp **grapeseed oil**

2 tbsp **tahini**

1 **garlic clove**, minced

4 **pitta breads**, split on one side

2 **plum tomatoes**, finely diced

25g (scant 1oz) **romaine lettuce**,
    thinly sliced

½ **red onion**, thinly sliced

1 In a small bowl, combine the ground flax seeds and 3 tablespoons of warm water. Set aside.

2 Heat 2 tablespoons of the olive oil in a small frying pan over a medium heat, until it shimmers (but before it begins to smoke). Add the onion, cumin, and coriander, and sauté, stirring constantly, for 5 minutes or until the onion softens and begins to brown.

3 Stir in the salt, black pepper, lemon zest, and 2 tablespoons of lemon juice. Remove from the heat, and stir in the coriander and flat-leaf parsley.

4 In a food processor fitted with a metal blade, process the chickpeas, breadcrumbs, and onion mixture for 1 minute or until chunky. Reserve 4 tablespoons of the mixture. Continue to process, adding the flax mixture, the remaining olive oil, and the reserved liquid from the chickpeas, until smooth. Pulse in the reserved chickpea mixture in 1 or 2 pulses, to evenly distribute. Divide the mixture into 8 evenly sized burgers 7.5cm (3in) wide and about 2.5cm (1in) thick.

5 In a large non-stick frying pan over a medium–high heat, heat the grapeseed oil. Add the falafel "burgers", and cook, turning once, until both sides are golden brown and the falafels are heated through.

6 In a small bowl, whisk together the tahini, garlic, and remaining lemon juice. Add 1 or 2 tablespoons of warm water, or enough to make a smooth dressing.

7 Fill each pitta with 2 falafel burgers and evenly divide the plum tomatoes, romaine lettuce, and red onion between the pittas. Drizzle the pittas with the tahini mixture, and serve immediately.

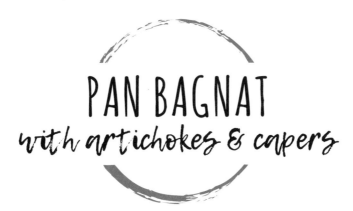

PAN BAGNAT
with artichokes & capers

MAKES 4
PREP 20 MINS

400g (14oz) can **chickpeas**, rinsed and drained

170g (6oz) jar marinated grilled **artichoke hearts**, drained, 2 tbsp marinade reserved

1 tbsp **salted capers**, rinsed and drained

1 tbsp **red wine vinegar**

1 tsp **dulse flakes**

4 crusty round **wholemeal rolls**, sliced

2 large **tomatoes**, sliced

4 leaves **romaine lettuce**

½ small **red onion**, sliced paper thin

2 tbsp chopped, pitted **black olives**

4 tbsp **extra virgin olive oil**

½ tsp freshly ground **black pepper**

1 In a food processor fitted with a metal blade, pulse the chickpeas, artichoke hearts, reserved artichoke heart marinade, capers, red wine vinegar, and dulse flakes until a rough, chunky purée consistency is reached.

2 Divide the chickpea mixture equally among the rolls. Top with tomato slices, romaine lettuce, and red onion slices.

3 Sprinkle the olives over the vegetables, drizzle each sandwich with a tablespoon of olive oil, and season liberally with black pepper. Serve with plenty of napkins!

VARIATION

For a variation, top the bread with wild rocket leaves, griddled aubergine slices, and finely sliced red onion. Then scatter over chopped green olives, and finish with a drizzle of chilli oil.

the good stuff

Dulse is a good source of potassium and iron, and rich in iodine and vitamin B6; it is invaluable for a plant-based diet.

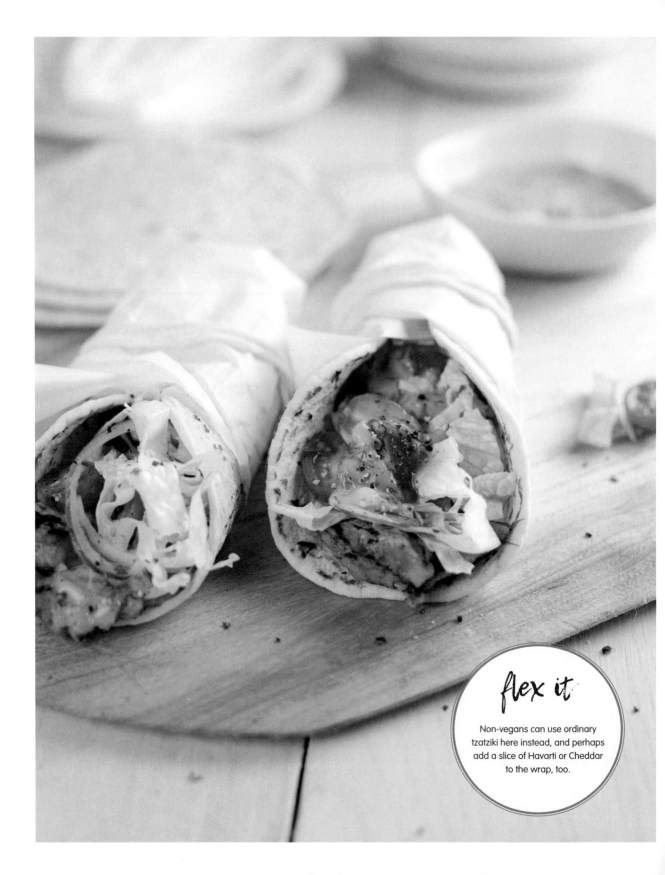

flex it

Non-vegans can use ordinary tzatziki here instead, and perhaps add a slice of Havarti or Cheddar to the wrap, too.

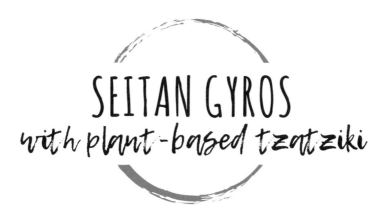

SEITAN GYROS
with plant-based tzatziki

MAKES 6
PREP 30 MINS
COOK 10 MINS

4 tbsp **extra virgin olive oil**,
   plus extra for grilling
juice of 2 **lemons**
2 tbsp finely chopped **flat-leaf**
   parsley
1 tsp **sea salt**
½ tsp freshly ground **black pepper**
1 **garlic clove**, crushed and
   finely chopped
1 loaf **seitan**
6 **pitta breads**
140g (5oz) shredded
   romaine lettuce
3 **plum tomatoes**, cored
   and cut into small dice
½ small **red onion**, very
   thinly sliced
plant-based tzatziki or 240ml
   (8fl oz) **plant-based yogurt** mixed
   with juice of ½ **lemon**
1 tsp **sweet paprika**

1 In a small bowl, whisk together the olive oil, lemon juice, flat-leaf parsley, salt, black pepper, and garlic.

2 Slice the seitan loaf very thinly and place the slices in a single layer in a large baking dish. Pour the marinade over the top and set aside at room temperature for 25 minutes.

3 Preheat a grill and brush the grill with a little olive oil.

4 Remove the seitan slices from the marinade, add to the grill, and grill for about 1 minute per side or until charred.

5 Quickly grill the pitta breads just to warm them. Evenly divide the seitan among the pitta, and top with romaine lettuce, plum tomatoes, and red onion. Drizzle each gyro with the plant-based tzatziki, sprinkle with sweet paprika, roll up, and serve immediately.

the good stuff

Seitan is a high-protein, low-calorie food – it is cholesterol-free and non-GMO, too. You can get your daily amount of riboflavin (B2) and B3 from 1 portion.

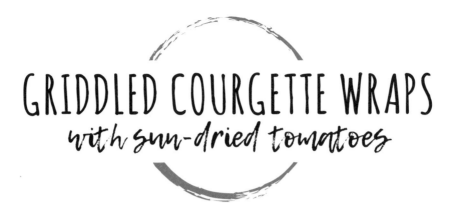

GRIDDLED COURGETTE WRAPS
with sun-dried tomatoes

SERVES 2
PREP 5 MINS
COOK 4–6 MINS

2 **courgettes**, cut into 5mm
   (¼in) slices lengthways
2 tbsp **olive oil**
2 large **flour tortillas**
6 tbsp **hummus**
8 **sun-dried tomatoes**
   in oil, drained and chopped,
   oil reserved
handful of **rocket**
lemon juice
freshly ground **black pepper**

1 Preheat a griddle pan. Brush the courgette slices with olive oil, then griddle for 2–3 minutes on each side or until tender and striped brown. Set aside.

2 Put the tortillas on a board and spread with the hummus. Lay the courgette strips on top and scatter with the sun-dried tomatoes.

3 Scatter the rocket on top, drizzle with the tomato oil and a squeeze of lemon juice, then add a good grinding of pepper. Fold in the sides, roll up each tightly, and cut in half.

the good stuff

Courgettes offer high levels of antioxidants and vitamin C. They also have anti-inflammatory properties. A protein-packed chickpea hummus is the perfect spread or dip for a vegan diet.

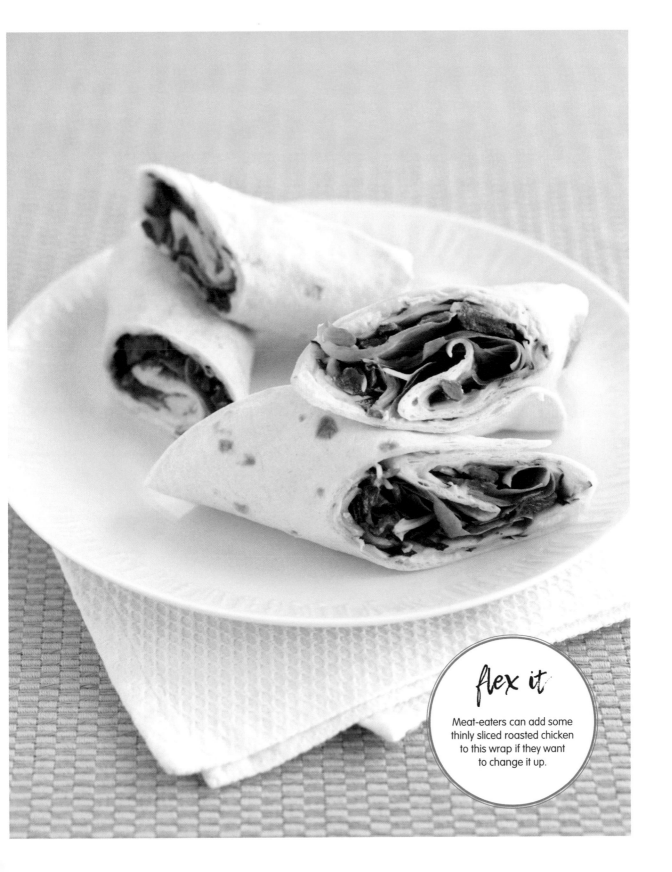

flex it

Meat-eaters can add some
thinly sliced roasted chicken
to this wrap if they want
to change it up.

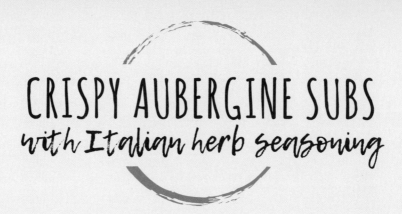

CRISPY AUBERGINE SUBS
with Italian herb seasoning

MAKES 4
PREP 15 MINS
COOK 15 MINS, plus draining

½ tsp **sea salt**
1 large **aubergine**, sliced
  lengthways in 5mm (¼in) slices
60g (2oz) **plain flour**
60g (2oz) **breadcrumbs**
2 tbsp **Italian herb seasoning**
1 tsp **garlic salt**
2 tbsp **olive oil**, plus extra olive oil
  or **grapeseed oil,** for frying
4 x 15cm (6in) **sub rolls**,
  sliced horizontally
1 **garlic clove**, halved
2 **tomatoes**, sliced
140g (5oz) **romaine** or **iceberg**
  lettuce, shredded
½ small **red onion**, sliced
  paper thin
hot peppadew peppers, drained
  and sliced (optional)
2 tbsp **red wine vinegar**

1 Sprinkle the salt over the aubergine slices, place these in a colander, and set aside to drain for 10 minutes. Pat the slices dry, squeezing gently to remove any bitter liquid.

2 In 3 separate shallow bowls, place 120ml (4fl oz) of water; the flour; the breadcrumbs, Italian herb seasoning, and garlic salt.

3 Coat the aubergine slices in the following manner: dip each slice first in the water, then in the flour, quickly dip in the water again, followed by the breadcrumbs. Dredge one last time in flour, and shake off any excess. Set aside each breaded slice, and continue until all slices are coated in this way.

4 In a large frying pan over medium–high heat, heat enough olive oil (or grapeseed oil) to come 5mm (¼in) up the side of the pan for shallow frying. When the oil shimmers, add the aubergine slices a few at a time, taking care not to crowd the pan. Fry for about 2 minutes or until golden and crispy, turn over the slices and fry the other side until golden. Set the cooked slices aside on a kitchen-paper-lined baking sheet, and repeat until all the aubergine has been fried.

5 Heat a grill to high, place the split sub rolls on a baking sheet, and toast for 2–3 minutes or until golden. Rub the toasted rolls with the cut garlic clove, and drizzle them evenly with the 2 tablespoons of olive oil.

6 To assemble the sandwiches, evenly divide the aubergine slices among the rolls. Top with the tomato, shredded lettuce, and red onion slices, again evenly distributing the ingredients. Place a few hot pepper slices (if using) on each sandwich, drizzle with the red wine vinegar, and serve.

OYSTER MUSHROOM PO'BOYS
with plant-based mayonnaise dressing

MAKES 4
PREP 15 MINS
COOK 5 MINS

4 tbsp **plant-based mayonnaise**
1 tbsp **tomato ketchup**
1 tbsp grated **sweet onion**
1 tbsp **pickled cucumber relish**
1 tsp finely chopped **chives**
125g (4½oz) **plain flour**
150g (5½oz) **fine polenta**
  (or cornmeal)
340g (¾ lb) **oyster mushrooms**,
  pulled apart into chunks
grapeseed oil, for frying
1 tsp **Old Bay seasoning**
½ tsp **sweet paprika**
4 x 15cm (6in) soft **sub rolls** (vegan),
  sliced horizontally
140g (5oz) **iceberg lettuce**,
  shredded
lemon wedges, to serve

1 In a small bowl, make the dressing by combining the plant-based mayonnaise, ketchup, grated onion, relish, and chives. Refrigerate until ready to use (this dressing can be made up to 3 days in advance).

2 In 3 separate shallow bowls, place 120ml (4fl oz) of water, flour, and polenta.

3 Coat the oyster mushrooms as follows: dip each first in the water, then in the flour, quickly dip in the water again, and then dredge thoroughly in polenta. Set aside each mushroom, and continue until all the mushrooms are coated in this way.

4 In a large frying pan over a medium heat, heat enough grapeseed oil to come 2cm (¾in) up the sides of the pan.

5 Add the breaded mushrooms to the frying pan, and fry for about 3 minutes, turning once or twice, until golden on all sides. Drain on kitchen paper, and sprinkle with Old Bay seasoning and sweet paprika.

6 Pile the mushrooms generously onto the sub rolls, drizzle each sandwich with about 1 tablespoon of dressing, top with the iceberg lettuce, and serve the lemon wedges on the side.

the good stuff

Oyster mushrooms provide the B vitamins riboflavin and niacin, which are especially important for people who don't eat meat. They are also a good source of selenium and potassium.

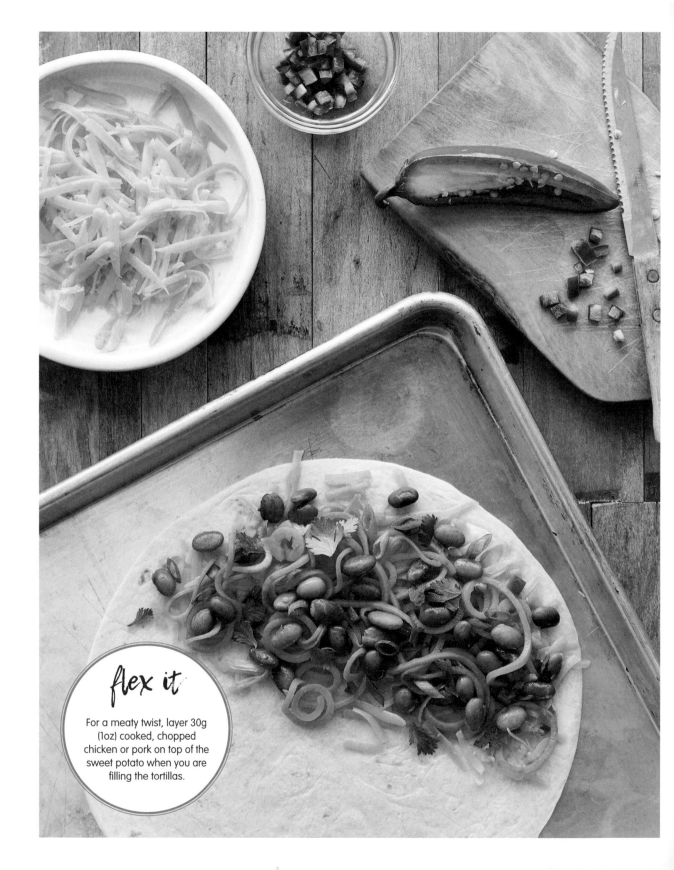

flex it

For a meaty twist, layer 30g (1oz) cooked, chopped chicken or pork on top of the sweet potato when you are filling the tortillas.

QUESADILLAS
with pinto beans & sweet potato

MAKES 4
PREP 20 MINS
COOK 40 MINS

1 small **sweet potato**, peeled
2 tbsp **vegetable oil**
1 **jalapeño chilli**, deseeded
   and diced
4 large **flour tortillas**
225g (8oz) finely grated
   **plant-based Cheddar-style
   cheese**
200g (7oz) cooked **pinto** or
   borlotti beans
45g (1½oz) chopped
   spring onion
15g (½oz) chopped
   coriander leaves
plant-based soured cream,
   to serve

1 With the medium blade of a spiralizer, spiralize the sweet potato.

2 In a medium frying pan, heat the vegetable oil over a medium–low heat until shimmering. Add the jalapeño and cook for 3 minutes, or until tender but not brown. Add the sweet potato and cook for 7 minutes, or until just al dente.

3 To assemble, place 1 tortilla on a clean, flat surface. Sprinkle about 28g (1oz) of the plant-based cheese on the lower half of the tortilla. Top with a quarter of the pinto beans and a quarter of the sweet potato. Add 2 tablespoons of onion and 2 tablespoons of coriander. Top with another 28g (1oz) cheese, then fold over the top of the tortilla to create a semicircle. Repeat to make 4 quesadillas in total.

4 Heat a non-stick frying pan over a medium heat. Add 1 quesadilla and cook for 4 minutes. Carefully turn, cover, and cook for another 4 minutes, until the tortilla is golden and the cheese melted. Repeat for the remaining 3 quesadillas.

5 Cut each quesadilla into 4 sections. Serve immediately with plant-based soured cream on the side.

the good stuff

Sweet potatoes are packed with vitamin C, potassium, and calcium. They also contain a load of beta-carotene, which helps reduce the appearance of ageing due to the powerful antioxidants in carotenoids.

PASTA & NOODLES

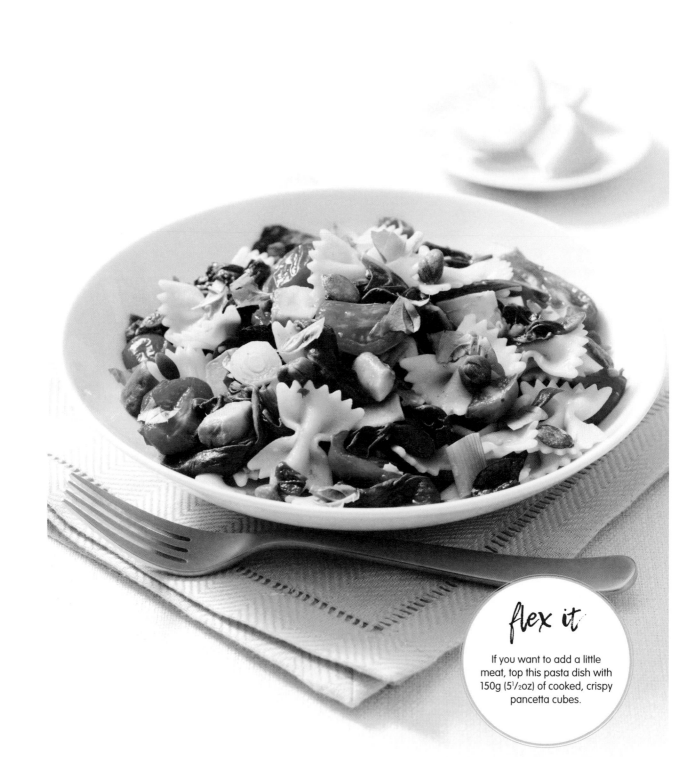

flex it

If you want to add a little meat, top this pasta dish with 150g (5½oz) of cooked, crispy pancetta cubes.

FARFALLE
with spinach, avocado, & tomatoes

SERVES 4
PREP 10 MINS
COOK 20 MINS

400g (14oz) **egg-free farfalle**

2 tbsp **olive oil**

4 **spring onions**, cut into
  short lengths

1 **garlic clove**, finely chopped

1 tsp **crushed dried chillies**

350g (12oz) **baby
  spinach leaves**

150ml (5fl oz) **vegetable stock**

4 **slow-roasted
  tomatoes**, chopped

175g (6oz) **baby plum
  tomatoes**, halved

30g (1oz) **black olives,**
  pitted and sliced

1½ tbsp **pickled capers**

2 **avocados**, diced

squeeze of **lemon juice**

salt and freshly ground
  black pepper

3 tbsp **pumpkin seeds**

lemon wedges, to garnish

torn **basil leaves**, to garnish

1 Cook the pasta according to the packet instructions, then drain. Heat the olive oil in a deep-sided sauté pan or wok. Add the spring onions and garlic and fry, stirring gently, for 1 minute. Stir in the chillies.

2 Add the spinach and stock and simmer, turning over gently for about 2 minutes until beginning to wilt. Gently fold in the pasta and the remaining ingredients. Simmer for 3 minutes until most of the liquid has been absorbed.

3 Pile into warmed, shallow bowls. Garnish with lemon wedges and a few torn basil leaves.

the good stuff

Spinach has outstanding health benefits, it is full of carotenoids and vitamin K. Thanks to its high levels of thylakoid, it can also help you curb hunger cravings.

CREAMY PASTA
with swiss chard & tomatoes

SERVES 4
PREP 5 MINS
COOK 15 MINS

450g (1lb) **egg-free fettuccine**
4 tbsp **extra virgin olive oil**
3 **garlic cloves**, thinly sliced
bunch of **Swiss chard**, washed well
   and torn into small pieces
½ tsp **sea salt**
2 large **tomatoes**, cored,
   deseeded, and cut into
   5mm (¼in) strips
8 tbsp **plant-based soured cream**
½ tsp **crushed chillies**

1 Cook the fettuccine in boiling, well-salted water according to the packet instructions.

2 Meanwhile, heat the olive oil in a large frying pan over a medium heat. Add the garlic and cook, stirring, for 30 seconds.

3 Add the Swiss chard and salt, and cook, stirring once or twice or until tender. Remove from the heat and cover to keep warm while the pasta finishes cooking.

4 When the pasta is ready, reserve 120ml (4fl oz) cooking water, and drain the pasta. Add the pasta to the Swiss chard along with the tomatoes, plant-based soured cream, and crushed chillies. Toss well, adding a little reserved pasta water, if needed, and serve immediately.

the good stuff

Swiss chard is another dark green leafy veg that should be included in a vegan diet as it is chock full of vitamins C, A, K, and B6, and important minerals, such as magnesium, iron, manganese, copper, and potassium.

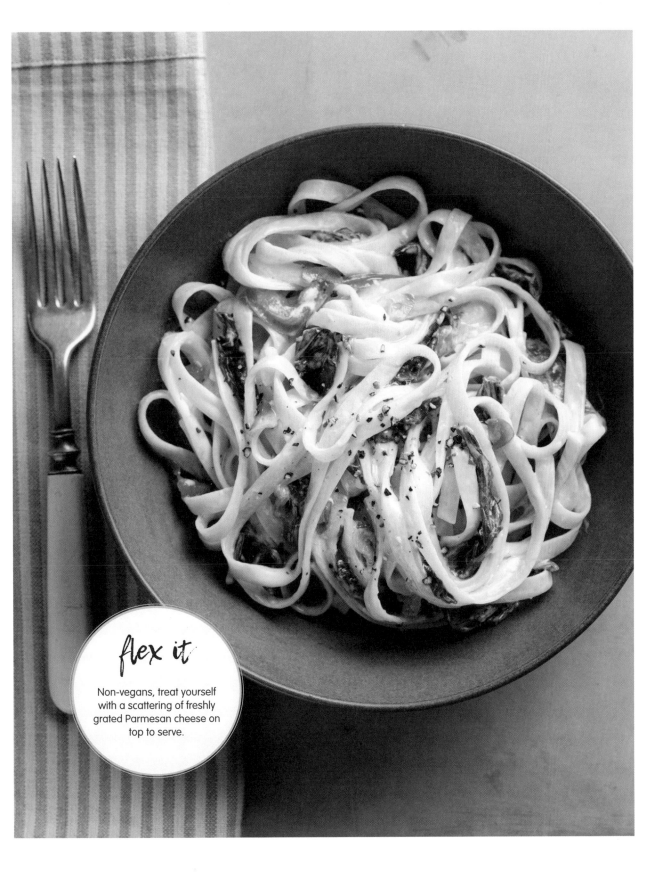

flex it

Non-vegans, treat yourself
with a scattering of freshly
grated Parmesan cheese on
top to serve.

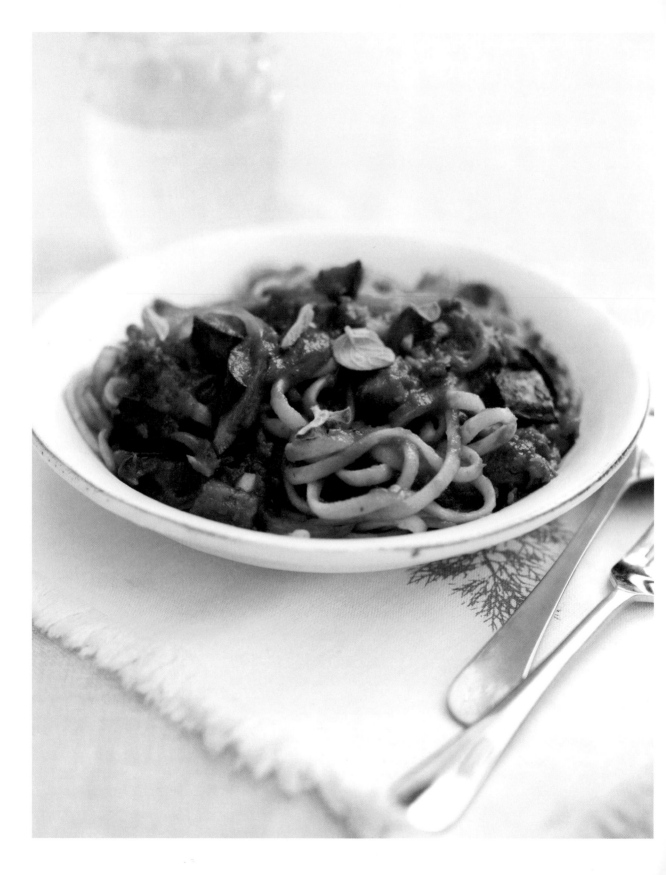

SPICED AUBERGINE LINGUINE
with chilli & oregano

SERVES 4
PREP 15 MINS
COOK 25 MINS

6 tbsp **olive oil**

2 **onions**, peeled and
finely chopped

2 **aubergines**, 1 cut into 1cm
(½in) dice, the other grated

4 **garlic cloves**, peeled
and chopped

½ tsp **chilli flakes**

500ml (16fl oz) **passata**

1 tsp **dried oregano**

salt and freshly ground
black pepper

400g (14oz) **egg-free linguine**

1 Pour the olive oil into a large frying pan and heat, add the onion and cook over a low heat for 3 minutes until soft, then add the diced aubergine and cook for 3 minutes more. Add the grated aubergine, garlic, and chilli flakes and cook for a further 3 minutes. Pour in the passata, add the oregano, and season well with salt and pepper. Bring to a simmer and allow to cook, uncovered, for 15 minutes.

2 Meanwhile add the pasta to a large pan of boiling salted water and cook for 8–10 minutes, or according to packet instructions. Drain and return to the pan.

3 Add half the aubergine mixture to the pasta and toss, then transfer to a large serving dish, or individual dishes, and top with the remaining sauce.

the good stuff

Garlic is a good way of adding flavour without piling on the salt. Aubergines contain an impressive array of vitamins and minerals, including high levels of fibre, folate, potassium, and manganese, as well as vitamins C, K, and B6, phosphorus, copper, thiamine, and magnesium.

VERMICELLI RICE NOODLES
with wasabi dressing

SERVES 2
PREP 15 MINS

70g (2¼oz) **dried vermicelli rice noodles**
75g (2½oz) **sugar snap peas**, finely sliced lengthways
4 **radishes**, finely sliced
finely grated zest of ½ **lime**, plus ½ **lime**, peeled, segmented, and chopped
1 tbsp **unsalted pistachio nuts**, roughly chopped
a few **basil leaves** (optional)
handful of **coriander leaves** (optional)
lime wedges (optional)

WASABI DRESSING
30g (1oz) **spinach leaves**
3 tbsp **silken tofu**
1 **garlic clove**, halved
juice of ½ **lemon**
sea salt and freshly ground **black pepper**
1–2 tsp **wasabi**, to taste

1 Put the vermicelli rice noodles in a bowl and cover with boiling water. Leave for 5 minutes (or according to the packet instructions), then drain, and set aside.

2 Meanwhile, make the dressing by putting the spinach leaves in a food processor and blending until chopped. Spoon in the silken tofu, add the garlic, lemon juice, and salt and pepper to taste, and blend again. Add the wasabi a little at a time, tasting and adding more wasabi or seasoning as needed, and blend until puréed. Spoon the dressing into a bowl. (This makes 4 servings. Store the extra servings in an airtight container in the fridge for up to 3 days.)

3 Mix the sugar snap peas, radishes, and lime zest in a bowl, season with salt and pepper, then toss with a little of the wasabi dressing.

4 Transfer the noodles to a serving bowl, then add the lime segments. Spoon in the sugar snap peas mixture and the remaining dressing, then sprinkle with the pistachios, basil, and coriander leaves (if using), and add the lime wedges (if using), to squeeze over the bowl.

the good stuff

Naturally sweet sugar snap peas are perfect for eating raw. They also make a good snack on their own as they are high in vitamin C and low in calories.

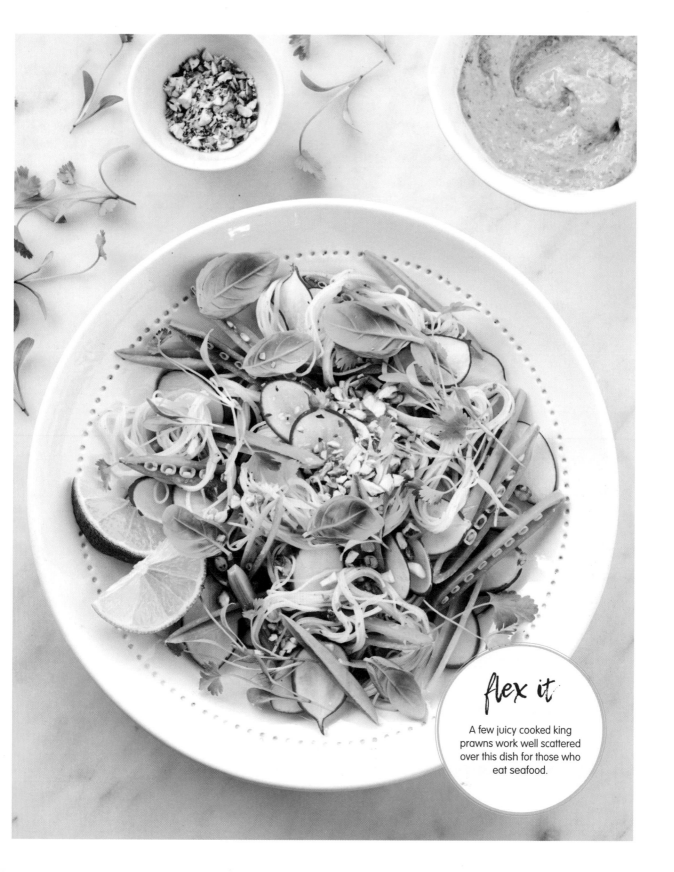

flex it

A few juicy cooked king prawns work well scattered over this dish for those who eat seafood.

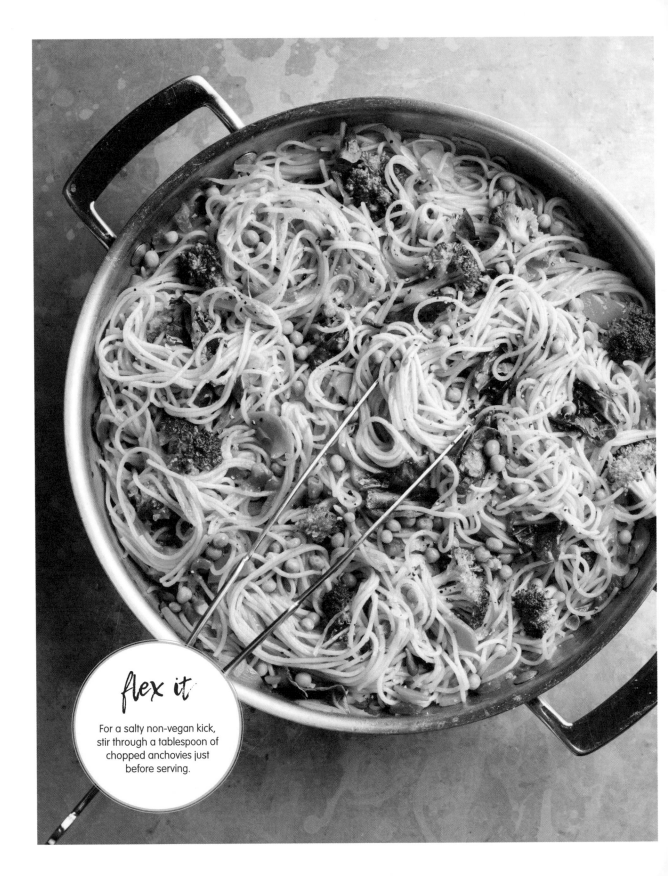

flex it

For a salty non-vegan kick,
stir through a tablespoon of
chopped anchovies just
before serving.

ONE-PAN PASTA PRIMAVERA
with broccoli, spinach, & peas

SERVES 4
PREP 10 MINS
COOK 20 MINS

4 tbsp **extra virgin olive oil**

1 **onion**, halved and thinly sliced

2 **garlic cloves**, thinly sliced

350g (12oz) **egg-free thin spaghetti**

1.1 litres (1¾ pints) **vegetable stock** or water

400g (14oz) can **chopped tomatoes**, with juice

140g (5oz) **fresh** or **frozen broccoli florets**

1 **carrot**, peeled, halved, and thinly sliced

1 tsp **sea salt**

140g (5oz) **baby spinach**

70g (2½oz) **fresh** or **frozen baby peas**

½ tsp freshly ground **black pepper**

1 Heat the olive oil in an extra-large frying pan with a lid over a medium–high heat. Add the onion and sauté for 2 minutes.

2 Add the garlic, spaghetti, vegetable stock, tomatoes with their juice, broccoli, carrot, and salt. Bring to the boil, reduce the heat to medium–low, cover, and cook for 3 minutes.

3 Uncover, stir, and continue cooking, stirring constantly and adjusting the heat as necessary to maintain a brisk simmer, for about 8 minutes or until the stock is absorbed and the pasta is tender.

4 Stir in the baby spinach, peas, and black pepper, toss for 1 minute, and serve immediately.

the good stuff

The greater the variety of vegetables you eat, the better for your health. Here you get your 5-a-day with a load of vitamin-rich veggies in one pan.

RAINBOW LENTIL MEATBALLS
with arrabiatta sauce

SERVES 4
PREP 20 MINS
COOK 45 MINS

300g (10oz) cooked **red lentils**,
   thoroughly drained
85g (3oz) cooked **brown lentils**,
   thoroughly drained
3 tbsp **aquafaba**, lightly beaten
45g (1½oz) **panko breadcrumbs**
½ tsp **garlic powder**
1 tsp **dried oregano**
zest of 1 large **lemon**
¼ tsp ground **cayenne pepper**
400g (14oz) **egg-free spaghetti**
plant-based Parmesan cheese,
   to serve (optional)

ARRABIATTA SAUCE
2 tbsp **olive oil**
1 small **onion**, finely chopped
2 x 400g (14oz) can
   chopped tomatoes
1 tbsp crushed **dried chillies**
salt and freshly ground
   black pepper

1 Preheat the oven to 180°C (350°F/Gas 4). Lightly oil a baking tray. In a large mixing bowl, combine the red lentils, brown lentils, aquafaba, breadcrumbs, garlic powder, oregano, lemon zest, and cayenne.

2 With your hands, form approximately 1 tablespoon of the lentil mixture into a meatball and place on the baking tray. Repeat with the remaining mixture. Bake for 25 minutes, rotating the meatballs halfway through.

3 Meanwhile, to make the arrabiatta sauce, in a saucepan warm the olive oil over a medium–low heat. Add the onion and cook for 2 minutes, or until soft. Add the tomatoes and chillies. Simmer over a low heat for 15 minutes, or until the sauce is warmed through. Season with salt and pepper to taste.

4 While the sauce is simmering, add the pasta to a large pan of boiling salted water and cook for 8–10 minutes or according to packet instructions. Drain and return to the pan.

5 Place the pasta and meatballs on 4 plates, top with the sauce, and serve immediately. Sprinkle with plant-based Parmesan cheese, if you like.

the good stuff

This dish is loaded with protein and fibre from the health-busting lentils and vitamin C-rich canned tomatoes – both are a must for the vegan store cupboard.

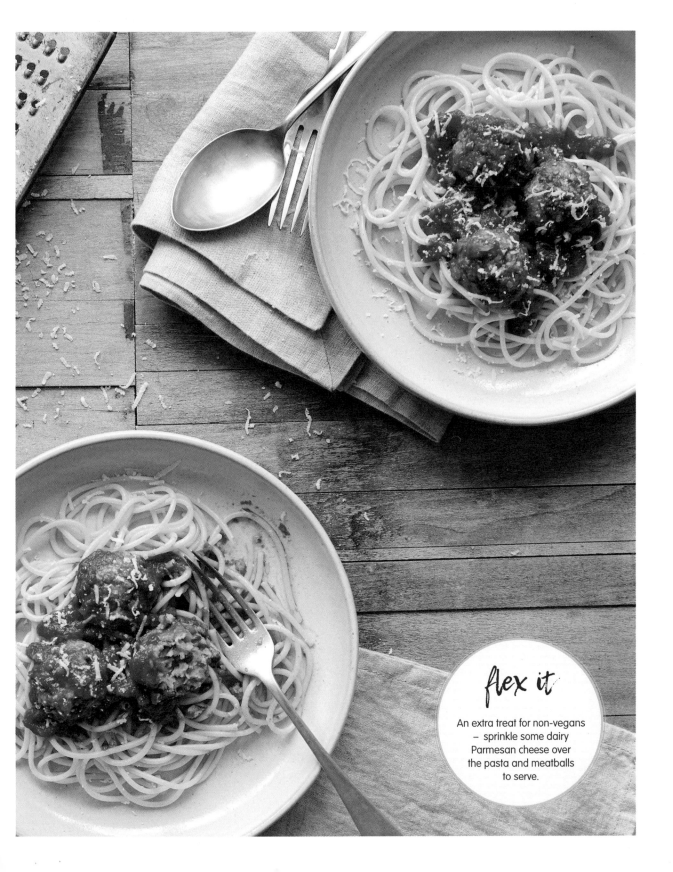

flex it

An extra treat for non-vegans – sprinkle some dairy Parmesan cheese over the pasta and meatballs to serve.

LEMON, GARLIC, & PARSLEY LINGUINE
with hot chilli flakes

SERVES 4
PREP 5 MINS
COOK 10 MINS

350g (12oz) **egg-free linguine**
3 tbsp **olive oil**
2 **garlic cloves**, finely chopped
zest of ½ **lemon** and juice of
  1 **lemon**
handful of **flat-leaf parsley**,
  finely chopped
pinch of **chilli flakes** (optional)
salt and freshly ground
  black pepper

1 Add the linguine to a large pan of salted boiling water and cook for 8–10 minutes or according to the instructions on the packet. Drain, then return to the pan with a little of the cooking water and toss together.

2 While the pasta is cooking, heat the olive oil in a frying pan, add the garlic and cook on a very low heat, being very careful not to burn it. Cook for about 1 minute, then add the lemon zest and juice and cook for a couple more minutes.

3 Stir in the parsley and chilli flakes, if using. Season with salt and black pepper then add the mixture to the pasta and toss to coat. A tomato and basil salad would work well with this dish.

the good stuff

Parsley not only acts as a flavour enhancer and garnish here, it is good to add to your food instead of salt, as it's full of vitamin K – a small bunch will provide almost all of your daily intake.

UDON NOODLES WITH SWEET & SOUR TOFU
& pickled ginger

SERVES 4
PREP 5 MINS
COOK 10 MINS

250g (9oz) **firm tofu**, cut into cubes
2 tbsp **sunflower oil**
1 tbsp **pickled ginger**
salt and freshly ground
   black pepper
300g (10oz) **egg-free udon**
   noodles

SWEET & SOUR SAUCE
1 tbsp **sunflower oil**
3 **garlic cloves**, finely chopped
5cm (2in) piece of **fresh root**
   ginger, cut into fine strips
pinch of **brown sugar**
10 **cherry tomatoes**, halved
4 **spring onions**, finely chopped
1 tbsp **dark soy sauce**
1 tbsp **rice vinegar**
1 tbsp **Chinese cooking wine**

1. First, make the sauce. Pour 1 tablespoon of sunflower oil into a wok, then add the garlic and fresh ginger and cook for 1 minute. Tip in the sugar and stir for a few seconds, then add the tomatoes and spring onions. Keep stirring for a few more minutes, until the tomatoes start to break down (you can squash them with the back of a fork).

2. Add the soy sauce, vinegar, and cooking wine. Bring to the boil, reduce to a simmer and cook for a couple of minutes.

3. Fry the tofu in 2 tablespoons of sunflower oil until golden. Stir the tofu and pickled ginger into the sweet and sour sauce. Taste, and season with salt and black pepper if required.

4. To finish, stir in the noodles and wait until they soften (about 2 minutes), then serve.

flex it

For the meat-eaters, swap the tofu for 250g (9oz) pork tenderloin, finely sliced, and fry it separately with the ingredients as you would the tofu.

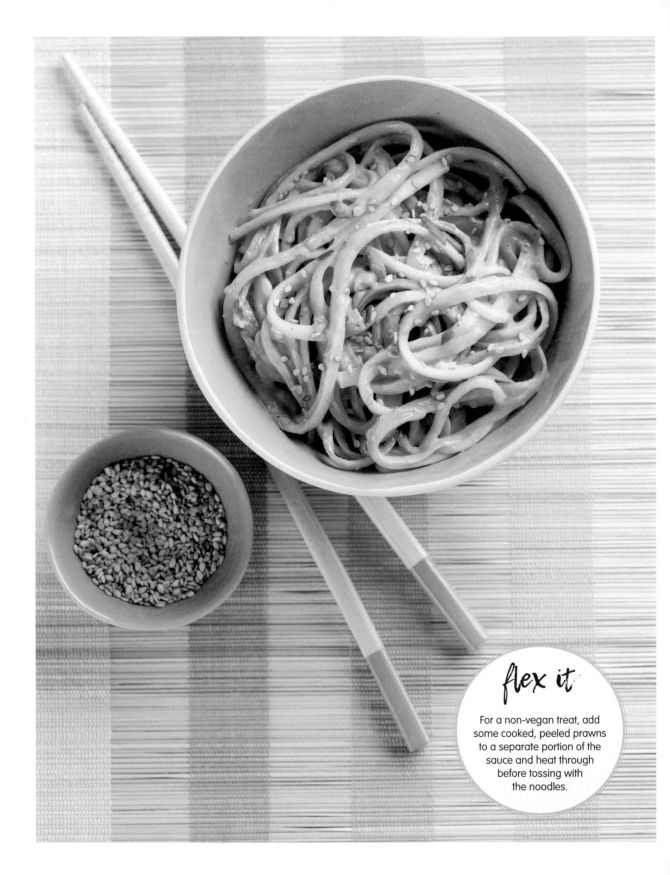

flex it

For a non-vegan treat, add some cooked, peeled prawns to a separate portion of the sauce and heat through before tossing with the noodles.

SESAME NOODLES
with peanut butter & tahini

SERVES 4
PREP 10 MINS
COOK 15 MINS

2 tsp **sea salt**
450g (1lb) **egg-free linguine**
4 tbsp **tahini**
4 tbsp **smooth peanut butter**
2 tbsp **low-sodium tamari**
  or **soy sauce**
2 tbsp **rice vinegar**
2 tbsp grated **fresh root ginger**
1 tsp **toasted sesame oil**
1 tsp **chilli garlic sauce**
1 **carrot**, julienned
1 **cucumber**, julienned
3 tbsp **gomasio**
4 tbsp thinly sliced **spring onions**,
  both light and dark green parts

1 Bring a large pan of water to the boil over a medium–high heat. Add the salt and linguine and cook for 8–10 minutes or according to the packet instructions until the pasta is tender. Drain, rinse the pasta under cold water, and set aside.

2 In a large bowl, whisk together the tahini, peanut butter, 4 tablespoons of hot water, tamari or soy sauce, rice vinegar, ginger, toasted sesame oil, and chilli garlic sauce.

3 Add the cooked linguine, carrot, and cucumber to the sauce. Toss gently, garnish with gomasio and spring onions, and serve immediately.

the good stuff

Tahini is a paste made from ground sesame seeds, and by using it you'll get most of your vitamins in one hit as it's high in vitamins E, B1, B2, B3, B5, and B15.

NO-COOK CRUNCHY STIR-FRY
with rice vinegar

SERVES 2
PREP 20 MINS

70g (2¼oz) **flat rice noodles**
135g (4¾oz) **carrot**, finely sliced
140g (5oz) **courgette**, finely sliced
½ **red pepper**, finely sliced
¼ **red chilli**, finely sliced
2 tsp **sesame seeds**
2.5cm (1in) piece of **lemongrass**,
  outer leaves removed, inner part
  finely sliced
60g (2oz) **button mushrooms**,
  halved
1 **spring onion**, trimmed, green
  part finely sliced, and white part
  sliced lengthways
a few **purple basil leaves** (optional)

DRESSING
1 tsp **dark soy sauce**
1 tsp **rice vinegar**
juice of ½ **lime**
½ **garlic clove**, grated
½ **red chilli**, finely chopped
sea salt and freshly ground
  black pepper

1 Put the rice noodles in a bowl and cover with boiling water. Leave for 10 minutes (or according to the packet instructions), then drain, and set aside.

2 Make the dressing by mixing the dark soy sauce, rice vinegar, lime juice, garlic, and red chilli in a bowl, and season with salt and pepper to taste.

3 Combine the carrot, courgette, red pepper, red chilli, sesame seeds, lemongrass, mushrooms, and the white part of the spring onion in a bowl. Add half the noodles and season with salt and pepper. Mix, trickle in the rice vinegar dressing, and mix again.

4 Transfer the no-cook stir-fry mix to a serving bowl, then add the remaining noodles. Sprinkle over the green part of the spring onion and the purple basil leaves (if using).

the good stuff

Eating your veg raw will ensure you get optimum nutrition, as none of the good stuff is lost in the cooking process.

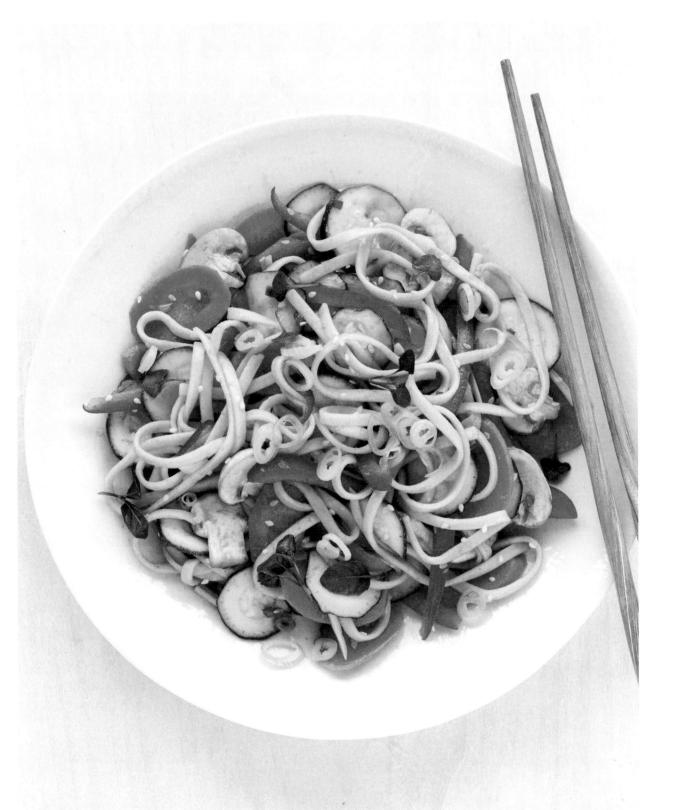

PULSES
& GRAINS

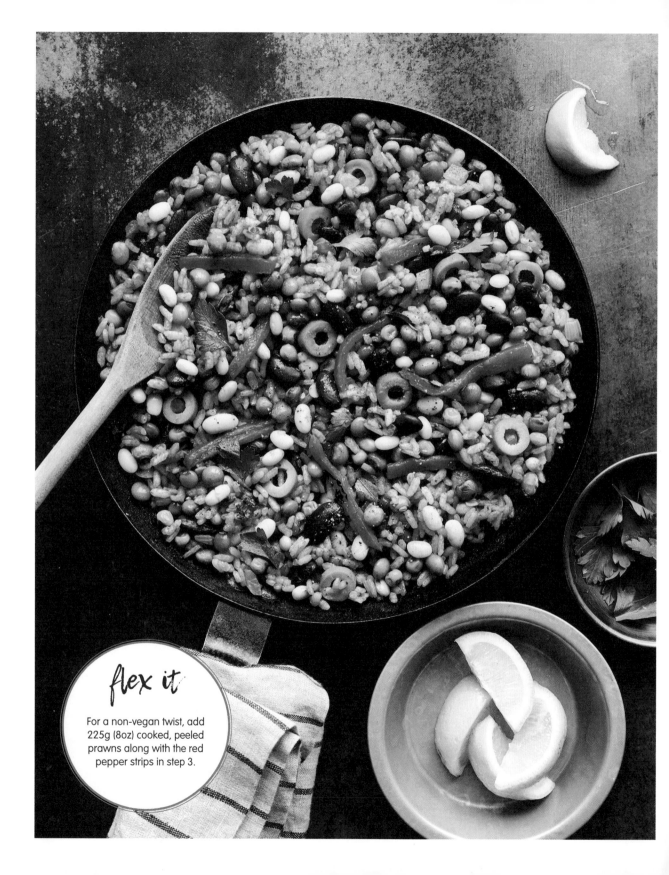

flex it

For a non-vegan twist, add 225g (8oz) cooked, peeled prawns along with the red pepper strips in step 3.

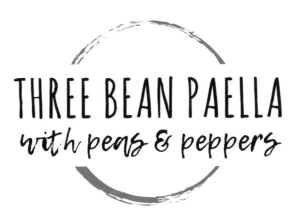

THREE BEAN PAELLA
with peas & peppers

SERVES 6
PREP 35 MINS
COOK 1 HR 5 MINS

2 tbsp **olive oil**
1 **onion**, chopped
3 **garlic cloves**, finely chopped
pinch of **saffron threads**
pinch of **crushed dried chillies**
225g (8oz) **chopped tomatoes**
1 tsp **smoked paprika**
450g (1lb) **paella rice**, such as
   Bomba or Calisparra
750ml (1¼ pints) **vegetable stock**
175g (6oz) cooked **haricot beans**
115g (4oz) cooked **pigeon peas**
   or **black-eyed beans**
125g (4½oz) cooked **kidney beans**
60g (2oz) **frozen peas**, thawed
salt and freshly ground
   black pepper
60g (2oz) **roasted red**
   pepper strips
60g (2oz) **green Spanish olives**,
   pitted and sliced
1 large **lemon**, cut into 8 wedges
flat-leaf parsley, to garnish

1 In a 25cm (10in) paella pan or large cast-iron frying pan, warm the olive oil over a medium heat until shimmering. Add the onion and cook for 2 minutes, or until it starts to soften. Stir in the garlic and cook for 30 seconds, or until fragrant. Incorporate the saffron, dried chillies, tomatoes, and paprika. Stir in the rice and cook for 2–3 minutes.

2 Add the stock to the rice mixture and stir. Bring to the boil then reduce the heat to low and cook, covered, for 20 minutes. Stir in the haricot beans, pigeon peas (or black-eyed beans), and kidney beans. Cover again and cook for an additional 10 minutes. Scatter the green peas across the top and cook without stirring, covered, for another 10 minutes, or until the beans and peas are warmed through. Remove from the heat.

3 Season with salt and pepper to taste. Arrange the red pepper strips and olives evenly across the top. Cover and let the paella stand for 5 minutes. Garnish with lemon wedges and parsley, then serve.

the good stuff

Only green veg comes as close to beans in value as a food source – it's important when eating a plant-based diet to aim to include beans most days.

ITALIAN TOMATO BARLEY RISOTTO
with green olives & basil

SERVES 4
PREP 10 MINS
COOK 45 MINS

1 tbsp **light olive oil**
1 **onion**, finely chopped
2 **garlic cloves**, crushed
300g (10oz) **pearl barley**, rinsed
375ml (13fl oz) **tomato passata**
600ml (1 pint) **vegetable stock**
1 tsp **Italian seasoning**
400g (14oz) can **cannellini beans**, drained
120g (4¼oz) **green olives**, pitted and halved
salt and freshly ground **black pepper**
handful of **basil leaves**, to garnish
plant-based Parmesan cheese, to serve (optional)

1 Heat the olive oil in a large, lidded saucepan over a medium-high heat. Add the onions and garlic and cook for about 5 minutes or until the onions are softened. Then add the barley to the pan, stir to coat with the oil, and cook for a further 2 minutes.

2 Add the passata, stock, and Italian seasoning to the pan. Stir well and reduce the heat to a simmer. Cover and cook for 30 minutes, or until most of the liquid has been absorbed and the barley is chewy. Make sure you stir the risotto occasionally to prevent the barley from sticking to the bottom of the pan.

3 Stir the beans into the risotto and cook for a further 5 minutes. Remove from the heat and stir in the olives, making sure they are evenly distributed. Season to taste, garnish with basil leaves, and serve hot. Serve with a bowl of plant-based Parmesan cheese to sprinkle over the top, if you like.

the good stuff

Barley is a fantastic plant-based source of protein – more so than brown rice – and fibre. It is also rich in magnesium and contains iron and vitamin B6.

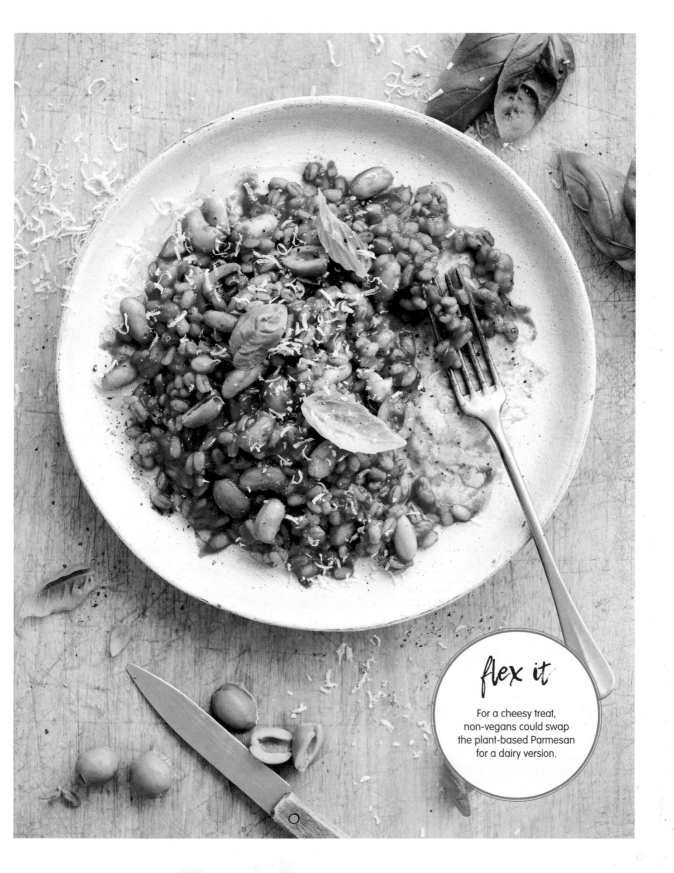

flex it

For a cheesy treat,
non-vegans could swap
the plant-based Parmesan
for a dairy version.

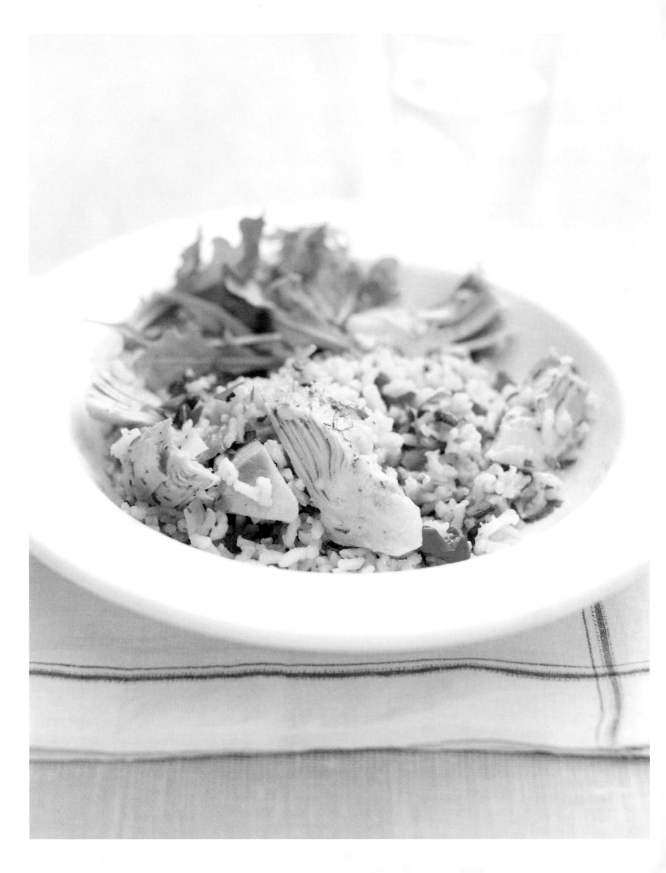

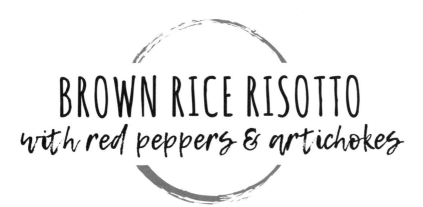

BROWN RICE RISOTTO
with red peppers & artichokes

SERVES 4
PREP 10 MINS
COOK 50 MINS–1 HR

1 tbsp **olive oil**
1 **onion**, finely chopped
salt and freshly ground
  black pepper
2 sweet **pointed red peppers**,
  halved, deseeded, and chopped
pinch of **chilli flakes**
280g (10oz) **brown rice**
1 litre (1¾ pints) **vegetable stock**
280g (10oz) jar of **artichoke hearts**,
  drained and roughly chopped
handful of **flat-leaf parsley**,
  finely chopped

1 Heat the olive oil in a large frying pan then add the onion and cook on a low heat until soft and transparent. Season with a pinch of salt and black pepper. Add the red peppers and cook for a few minutes until they soften.

2 Add the chilli flakes, then stir in the rice. Raise the heat a little, pour in a ladleful of the stock, and bring to the boil. Reduce to a simmer and cook gently for 40–50 minutes, adding a little more stock each time the liquid is absorbed, until the rice is cooked.

3 Stir through the artichokes and cook for a couple of minutes to heat through, then taste and season as required. Cover with a lid, remove from the heat and leave for 10 minutes, then stir through the chopped parsley and transfer to plates or bowls. You could serve this with a rocket salad on the side.

the good stuff

Just 225g (8oz) of brown rice provides heaps of your daily fibre requirement. It's an important grain for a plant-based diet as it is rich in protein, thiamine, calcium, magnesium, fibre, and potassium.

SWEET POTATO & SPINACH CURRY
with ginger & coriander

SERVES 4
PREP 10 MINS
COOK 20 MINS

2 tbsp **coconut oil**

1 **onion**, finely chopped

2 **garlic cloves**, crushed

5cm (2in) piece of **fresh root ginger**, grated

1 tsp **mustard seeds**

¼ tsp **ground cinnamon**

½ tsp **ground turmeric**

½ tsp **cayenne pepper**

1 tsp **ground cumin**

1 tsp **ground coriander**

400ml (14oz) can **reduced-fat coconut milk**

250ml (9fl oz) **vegetable stock**

3 large **sweet potatoes**, peeled and cut into 3cm (1½in) cubes, about 700g (25oz) in total

100g (3½oz) **baby spinach leaves**

salt, to taste

1 small handful of **coriander leaves**, roughly chopped

1 Heat the coconut oil in a large, shallow pan. Fry the onion over a medium heat for 3–4 minutes, until it has softened but is not brown. Add the garlic and ginger, and cook for a further minute, then add all the remaining spices and cook over a low heat for a further minute, stirring constantly, until they darken slightly and start to release their fragrance.

2 Add the coconut milk and vegetable stock to the pan and mix well. Add the diced sweet potatoes and bring the mixture to the boil, then reduce to a low simmer and cook, covered, for 10–12 minutes until the potatoes are just soft.

3 Remove the lid and gently stir in the spinach leaves to avoid breaking up the sweet potatoes. The curry is ready when the spinach has wilted into the sauce, which should take about 1–2 minutes. Taste and add a little salt, if needed.

4 Remove from the heat and stir in the chopped coriander before serving with cooked brown rice.

the good stuff

Sweet potatoes, spinach, and coconut milk make this a dish rich in vitamin C. It is flavoured with superfood spices, too – mustard seeds and turmeric have anti-inflammatory properties.

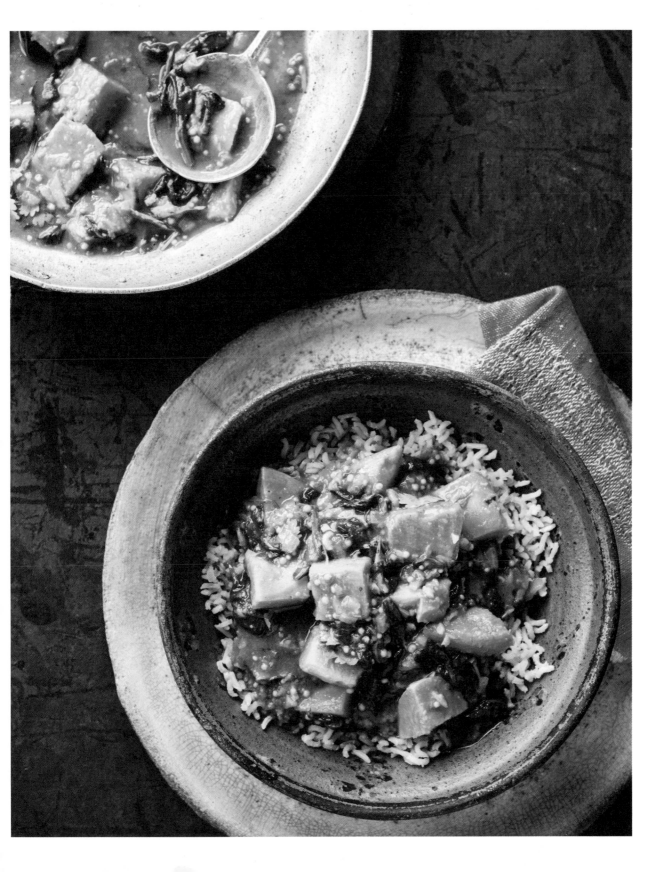

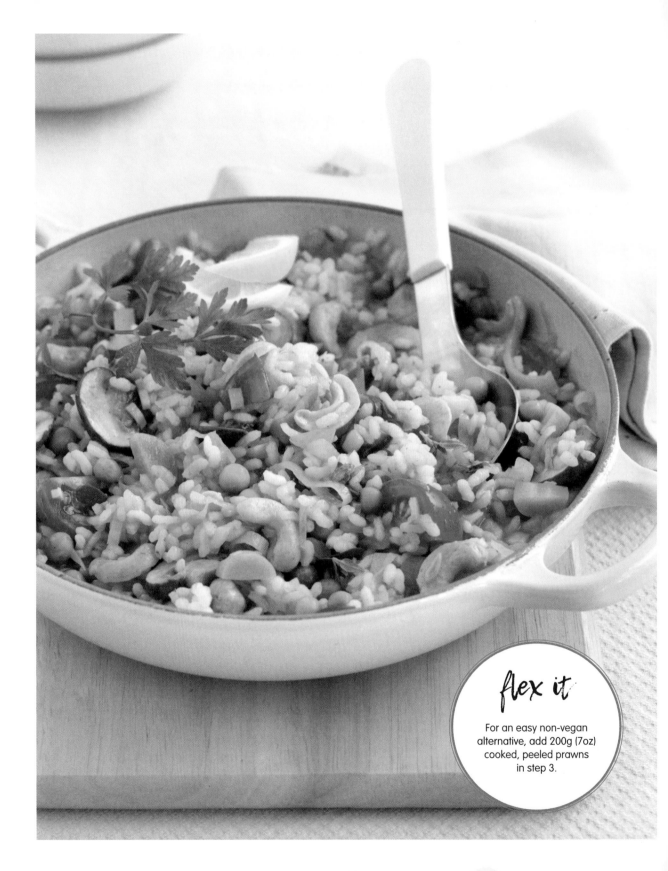

flex it

For an easy non-vegan alternative, add 200g (7oz) cooked, peeled prawns in step 3.

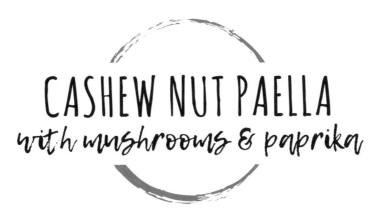

CASHEW NUT PAELLA
with mushrooms & paprika

SERVES 4
PREP 10 MINS
COOK 25 MINS

large pinch of **saffron strands**
750ml (1¼ pints) hot
  vegetable stock
2 tbsp **olive oil**
1 **leek**, chopped
1 **onion**, chopped
2 **garlic cloves**, crushed
1 **red pepper**, deseeded
  and chopped
1 **carrot**, chopped
250g (9oz) **paella rice**
150ml (5fl oz) **dry white wine**
115g (4oz) **chestnut**
  mushrooms, sliced
115g (4oz) **roasted, unsalted**
  cashew nuts
salt and freshly ground
  black pepper
115g (4oz) **fresh shelled**
  or **frozen peas**
1½ tbsp chopped **thyme**
4 **tomatoes**, quartered
½ tsp **smoked paprika**
sprig of **flat-leaf parsley**,
  to garnish
lemon wedges, to garnish

1 Put the saffron strands in the stock to infuse. Heat the olive oil in a paella pan or large frying pan and fry the leek, onion, garlic, red pepper, and carrot, stirring, for 3 minutes until softened, but not browned. Add the rice and stir until coated in oil and glistening.

2 Add the wine and boil until it has been absorbed, stirring. Stir in the saffron-infused stock, mushrooms, nuts, and some salt and pepper. Bring to the boil, stirring once, then reduce the heat, cover, and simmer very gently for 10 minutes.

3 Add the peas and thyme, stir gently, then distribute the tomatoes over the top. Cover and simmer very gently for a further 10 minutes until the rice is just tender and has absorbed most of the liquid, but is still creamy.

4 Sprinkle the paprika over and stir through gently, taking care not to break up the tomatoes. Taste and adjust the seasoning, if necessary.

5 Garnish with a sprig of parsley and lemon wedges and serve hot with crusty bread and a green salad.

the good stuff

Although good for you – cashews contain high levels of vitamin E, magnesium, and zinc – they are also fairly high in fat, so don't overindulge.

BUCKWHEAT STIR-FRY
with aubergine, courgette, & kale

SERVES 4
PREP 15 MINS
COOK 20 MINS

pinch of **salt**
175g (6oz) **buckwheat**
3 tbsp **grapeseed oil**
2 **dried red chillies**
1 **garlic clove**, thinly sliced
1 tsp grated **fresh root ginger**
drizzle of **toasted sesame
  oil** (optional)
4 **Japanese aubergines**, cut
  into cubes
2 **courgettes**, cut into cubes
4 **kale leaves**, ribs removed
  and roughly chopped
handful of **basil leaves**,
  roughly chopped
sesame seeds, to garnish

MISO
2 tbsp **white miso**
1½ tsp **brown rice vinegar**
1 tsp grated **fresh root ginger**

1 Place 500ml (16fl oz) of water in a large, lidded saucepan and add a pinch of salt. Bring to the boil, then slowly stir in the buckwheat. Reduce the heat to a simmer, cover, and cook for 15 minutes. Then remove from the heat, cover, and leave to stand.

2 Meanwhile, heat the grapeseed oil in a large frying pan over a medium heat. Add the chillies and cook for about 2 minutes, stirring, until fragrant. Add the garlic, ginger, and sesame oil, if using, and cook for 2 minutes, stirring frequently. Then add the aubergines and courgettes and cook for a further 8–10 minutes, stirring frequently, until the vegetables are cooked through.

3 Meanwhile, for the miso, place all the ingredients in a bowl, add 1 teaspoon of water, and mix until well combined. Stir the mixture into the vegetables and mix well to coat. Then add the kale and cook for a further 2–3 minutes, until just wilted. Remove from the heat and sprinkle over the basil and sesame seeds. Serve hot over the buckwheat.

the good stuff

This colourful dish introduces a variety of healthy veg such as kale, which is high in iron, as well as healthy and filling buckwheat, which is rich in manganese and magnesium.

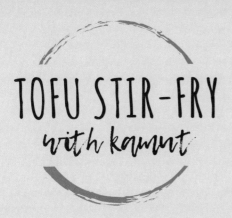

TOFU STIR-FRY
with kamut

SERVES 2
PREP 15 MINS, plus marinating and soaking
COOK 1 HR

400g (14oz) **firm tofu**, drained and cubed
100g (3½oz) **raw kamut**
3 tbsp **vegetable oil**
1 **carrot**, cut into sticks
1 **red pepper**, deseeded and thinly sliced
50g (1¾oz) **beansprouts**
4 **spring onions**, thinly sliced
salt and freshly ground **black pepper**

MARINADE
4 tbsp **soy sauce**
2 tbsp **maple syrup**
5cm (2in) piece of **fresh root ginger**, finely chopped
2 **garlic cloves**, finely chopped

1 Combine the marinade ingredients in a bowl. Place the tofu in a plastic bag along with half the marinade. Seal, and shake to coat. Marinate in the fridge for 3–4 hours. Reserve the marinade.

2 Place the kamut in a bowl, cover with water, and soak for 8 hours. Rinse and drain, then place in a lidded saucepan. Cover with water and bring to the boil. Simmer for 45 minutes or until tender. Drain.

3 Heat 2 tablespoons of oil in a frying pan over a medium–high heat. Sauté the tofu for 10 minutes, until browned. Remove with a slotted spoon. Add the remaining oil to the pan and cook the carrots and peppers for 2 minutes, stirring frequently. Then add the beansprouts and cook for 3 minutes, stirring. Stir in the kamut, tofu, and reserved marinade. Add the onions and cook for 2 minutes. Season to taste.

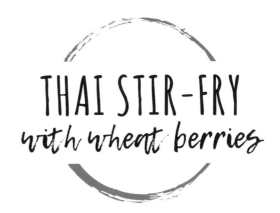

THAI STIR-FRY
with wheat berries

SERVES 2
PREP 10 MINS
COOK 1 HR

100g (3½oz) **wheat berries**
2 tbsp **smooth peanut butter**
2 tbsp **maple syrup**
1 tbsp **soy sauce**
¼ tsp **chilli flakes**
juice of 1 **lime**
1 tbsp **vegetable oil**
75g (2½oz) **beansprouts**
50g (1¾oz) **green cabbage**, shredded
1 **carrot**, sliced into matchsticks
100g (3½oz) **soya beans**
salt and freshly ground **black pepper**
2 tbsp roughly chopped **coriander leaves**

1 Place the wheat berries in a pan, cover with water, and bring to the boil. Reduce the heat to a simmer, cover, and cook for 45–50 minutes, until tender. Remove from the heat and drain any remaining water.

2 Place the peanut butter, maple syrup, soy sauce, and chilli flakes in a bowl and mix to combine. Then add the lime juice and mix until it forms a smooth sauce. Heat the vegetable oil in a large frying pan over a high heat. Add the beansprouts, cabbage, and carrots and stir-fry for 3–5 minutes. Then add the soya beans and wheat berries and stir-fry for a further 2 minutes. Pour over the peanut sauce and toss to coat. Season to taste and remove from the heat. Sprinkle with coriander and serve hot.

VEGETABLE STIR-FRY
with sprouted quinoa & sesame

SERVES 2
PREP 10 MINS
COOK 5 MINS

2 tbsp **vegetable oil**

2 tsp **sesame oil**

1 **carrot**, peeled and julienned

¼ **red onion**, finely sliced

½ **courgette**, julienned

60g (2oz) **sprouted mung beans**

60g (2oz) **Savoy cabbage**,
  finely shredded

2 tbsp finely chopped
  fresh root ginger

2 **garlic cloves**, crushed or
  finely chopped

1 **jalapeño** or **other chilli**,
  deseeded, and finely chopped

450g (1lb) **sprouted quinoa**

2 tbsp **sprouted sesame seeds**

2 tbsp **low-sodium soy sauce**

1 Heat a wok or large frying pan over a high heat and add the vegetable and sesame oils. When the oil has almost begun to smoke, add the carrot, and stir-fry for 1 minute. Add the onion and courgette and cook for another minute. Add the sprouted mung beans, cabbage, ginger, garlic, and jalapeño and cook for 1 minute more.

2 Add the sprouted quinoa and sesame seeds to the vegetables, and cook over a high heat, turning constantly, until the quinoa begins to brown, about 2 minutes. Add the soy sauce to the pan and cook for a final minute before serving immediately.

the good stuff

Sprouting may increase the grains' essential nutrients – an impressive list of B vitamins, vitamin C, folate, soluble fibre, and amino acids. As these sprouts are only lightly cooked, it's best to avoid serving this salad to children and pregnant women – raw sprouted seeds, grains, and pulses carry a risk of foodborne bacteria.

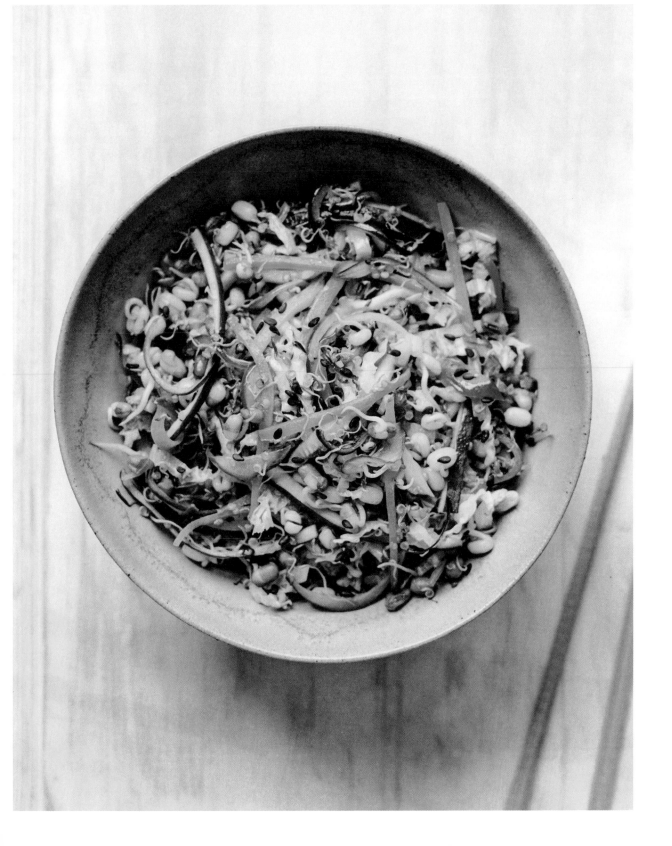

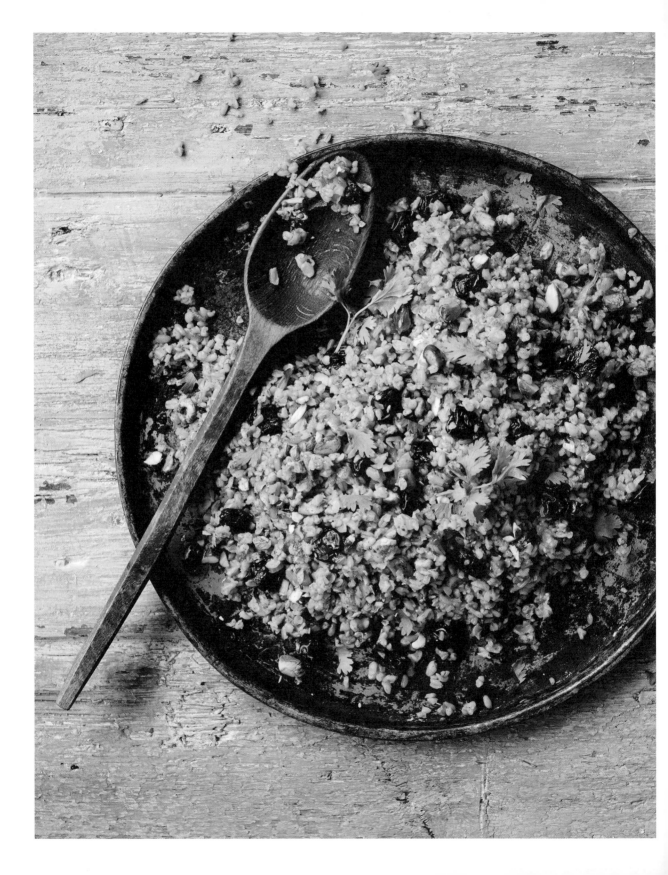

CHERRY & PISTACHIO FREEKEH PILAF
with lemon dressing

SERVES 4
PREP 5 MINS
COOK 20–25 MINS

200g (7oz) **freekeh**
8 **cardamom pods**
8 **whole cloves**
1 tbsp **olive oil**
1 **onion**, finely chopped
1 tsp **ground cinnamon**
pinch of **salt**
100g (3½oz) **dried cherries**,
  roughly chopped
100g (3½oz) **pistachio nuts**,
  roughly chopped

LEMON DRESSING
3 tbsp **olive oil**
2 tbsp **lemon juice**
pinch of **salt**

1 Place the freekeh in a large saucepan, cover with 1 litre (1¾ pints) of water, and place over a medium heat. Add the cardamom and cloves and simmer for 20 minutes or until all the water has been absorbed. Drain any remaining water, then remove and discard the cardamom pods and cloves. Set aside.

2 Meanwhile, heat the olive oil in a large frying pan over a medium heat. Add the onions to the pan and cook for 5–10 minutes, stirring occasionally, until softened and translucent. Then add the cinnamon and cook for a further 2 minutes.

3 For the lemon dressing, place all the ingredients in a small bowl and mix to combine.

4 Add the freekeh to the onion mixture, season with the salt, and stir to mix. Then add the cherries and pistachio nuts and stir until evenly distributed. Remove from the heat. Serve hot with the dressing drizzled over.

the good stuff

Adding dried cherries to your plant-based diet will increase your intake of copper and essential minerals.

ROASTED ROOTS & PULSES BOWL
with kale & walnuts

SERVES 2
PREP 15 MINS
COOK 40 MINS

100g (3½oz) **beetroot**
100g (3½oz) **carrot**
100g (3½oz) **celeriac**
100g (3½oz) **sweet potato**
1 tbsp **olive oil**
½ tsp **ground cumin**
salt and **pepper** to taste
85g (3oz) cooked **chickpeas**
1 **garlic clove**, crushed
pinch of **cayenne pepper**
30g (1oz) **puy lentils**
   or **green lentils**
25g (scant 1oz) **quinoa**, rinsed
20g (¾oz) **kale leaves**, chopped
10g (¼oz) **rocket**
1 tbsp **walnut pieces**
1 tsp **pumpkin seeds**

DRESSING
1 tbsp **olive oil**
1 tsp **wholegrain mustard**
2 tsp **maple syrup**

1 Preheat the oven to 180°C (350°F/Gas 4). Leaving the skins on, wash and chop the beetroot, carrot, celeriac, and sweet potato into equal-sized chunks. Place each of the 4 root vegetables in its own quarter of a large roasting tray and drizzle over ½ tablespoon of the olive oil. Sprinkle with cumin and season with salt and pepper.

2 Place the chickpeas in a roasting tray with the garlic and ½ tablespoon of olive oil. Season with salt, pepper, and the pinch of cayenne. Place both trays in the oven. Cook the chickpeas for 15 minutes and the root vegetables for 25 minutes.

3 Rinse the lentils and place in a pan. Cover with water and bring to the boil. Reduce the heat and simmer, covered, for 10 minutes. Add the quinoa and cook for 5 minutes. Steam the kale over the lentils and quinoa for 5 minutes, until it wilts. Drain the lentils and quinoa.

4 For the dressing, whisk up the olive oil, mustard, and maple syrup.

5 Layer up the lentils and quinoa, root vegetables, rocket, kale, and chickpeas in a bowl. Sprinkle with walnuts and pumpkin seeds, then drizzle with the dressing.

the good stuff

Root veggies are packed with vitamins, especially A and C, and should be included in a vegan diet, especially in the winter when our body craves vitamin C. They are also a good form of fibre.

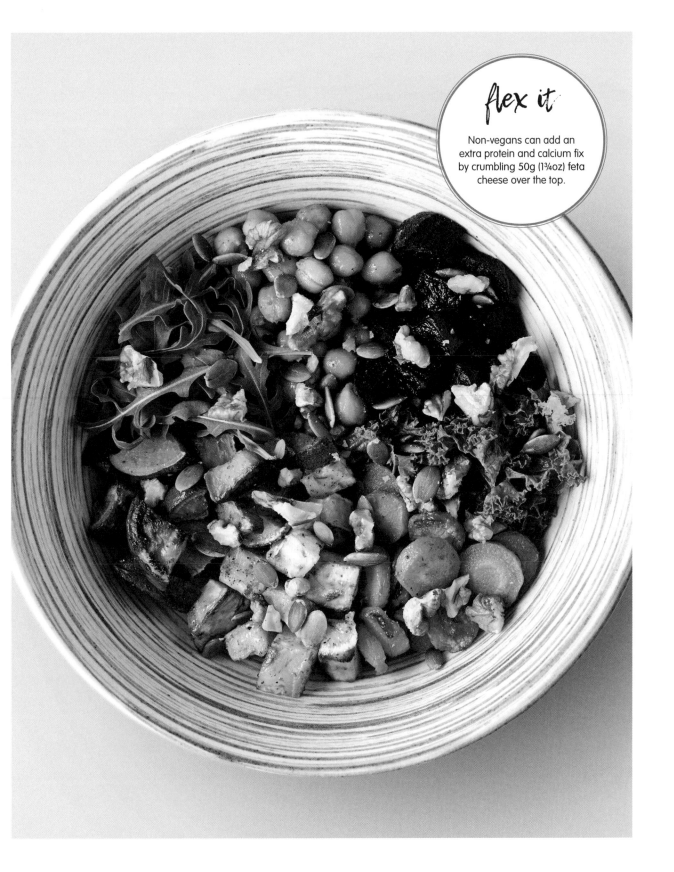

flex it

Non-vegans can add an extra protein and calcium fix by crumbling 50g (1¾oz) feta cheese over the top.

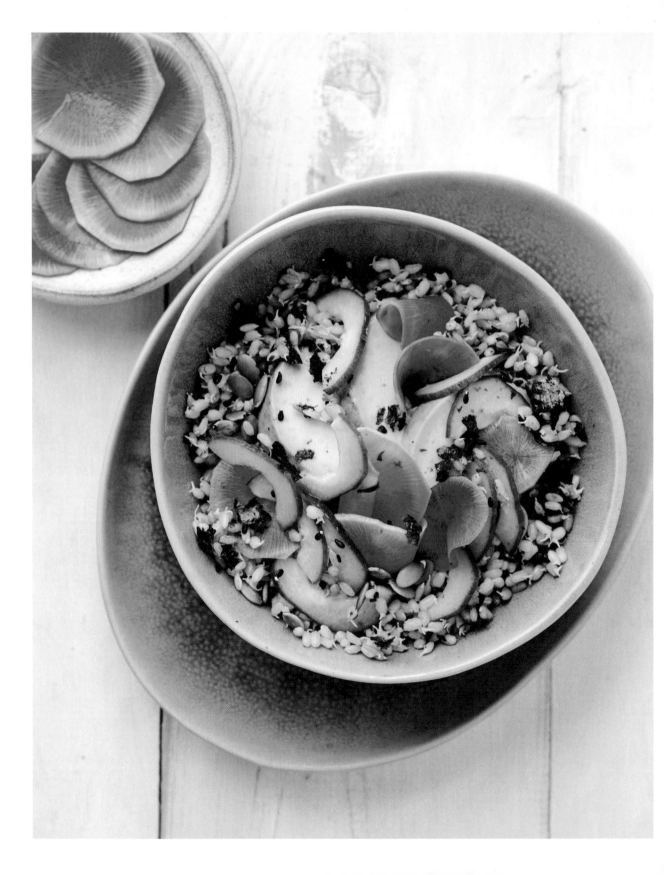

BROWN RICE SUSHI BOWL
with sprouted seeds & pickled radishes

SERVES 1
PREP 15 MINS, plus chilling
COOK 20 MINS

160g (5¾oz) **sprouted short-grain brown rice**
1 tbsp **rice wine vinegar**
¼ tsp **sugar**
¼ tsp **salt**
1 tbsp **sprouted pumpkin seeds**
1 tbsp **sprouted sunflower seeds**
1 tbsp **sprouted sesame seeds**
5g (⅕oz) **dried seaweed sheets**
2.5cm (1in) piece of **cucumber**, halved, deseeded, and finely sliced
½ **small avocado**, sliced

PICKLED RADISHES
120ml (4fl oz) **rice wine vinegar**
40g (1¼oz) **granulated sugar**
1 tsp **fine sea salt**
4 **watermelon radishes**, washed, trimmed, and finely sliced

1 To make the pickled radishes, whisk together the vinegar, sugar, and salt in a small bowl until the sugar has dissolved. Pack the radishes into a small Kilner or mason jar, pour the vinegar mixture over them until completely covered, and seal. Refrigerate for at least 1 hour before using. (These will keep in the refrigerator for up to 1 week.)

2 Place the sprouted brown rice in a medium heavy-based saucepan and cover with 240ml (8fl oz) of cold water. Bring to the boil, then reduce the heat to a simmer and cook, covered, for 15–20 minutes, until all the water has evaporated and the rice is nearly tender.

3 Put the vinegar, sugar, and salt in a small saucepan and heat, whisking, until the sugar is just dissolved. Mix the dressing into the rice and let it sit, covered, for 5 minutes.

4 Mix the sprouted pumpkin seeds, sunflower seeds, and sesame seeds into the warm rice. Set aside 1–2 of the seaweed sheets and crumble the rest over the rice. Mix well to combine.

5 Turn the warm rice mixture into a serving bowl and top it with the cucumber, avocado, and a few slices of the pickled radishes. Crumble the remaining seaweed sheets over the top and serve.

the good stuff

Seaweed is more nutrient-dense than any other land vegetable. It provides stacks of nutrients and a rich supply of minerals, mainly calcium – especially good for vegans as they exclude dairy.

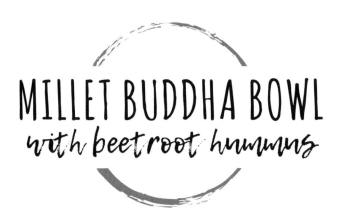

MILLET BUDDHA BOWL
with beetroot hummus

SERVES 1
PREP 15 MINS, plus soaking
COOK 45 MINS

50g (1¾oz) **millet**
1 **corn on the cob**
small handful of **baby spinach**
handful of **pea shoots** or **baby salad leaves**
50g (1¾oz) cooked **cannellini beans**
2 **chestnut mushrooms**, sliced
1 small **carrot**, julienned or grated
½ small **mango**, peeled and diced
1 tbsp **sunflower seeds**
2 **lime** wedges, to garnish

BEETROOT HUMMUS
100g (3½oz) **beetroot**, roughly chopped
½ tbsp **olive oil**, plus extra for drizzling
juice of ½ **lemon**
salt and freshly ground **black pepper**

DRESSING
1 tbsp **olive oil**
2 tsp **balsamic vinegar**

1 Soak the millet overnight in double the volume of water. Drain and rinse well.

2 For the beetroot hummus, preheat the oven to 180°C (350°F/Gas 4). Place the beetroot in a roasting tray, drizzle with some oil and roast for 30 minutes until soft. Then add to a blender and whizz. With the motor running, drizzle in the olive oil, and add 1–3 tablespoons of water until the desired consistency is reached. Season to taste with lemon, salt, and pepper.

3 Place the millet in a small saucepan, cover with water and bring to the boil. Lower the heat and simmer for 10 minutes until soft but not mushy. Drain and place in a mixing bowl.

4 Using a sharp knife, slice the corn kernels off the cob and combine with the cooked millet.

5 To make the dressing, combine the olive oil and vinegar in a small dish or glass jar and shake well.

6 Put a bed of millet and sweetcorn in a bowl and arrange the greens, beans, vegetables, and mango around it with a generous dollop of beetroot hummus in the middle.

7 Drizzle with the dressing, sprinkle with sunflower seeds, and garnish with lime wedges. Season with salt and pepper.

the good stuff

It's hard to beat beetroot as a healthy food; it's rich in nitrates, vitamin C, and iron, and a great source of lysine – an essential amino acid that your body can't produce on its own.

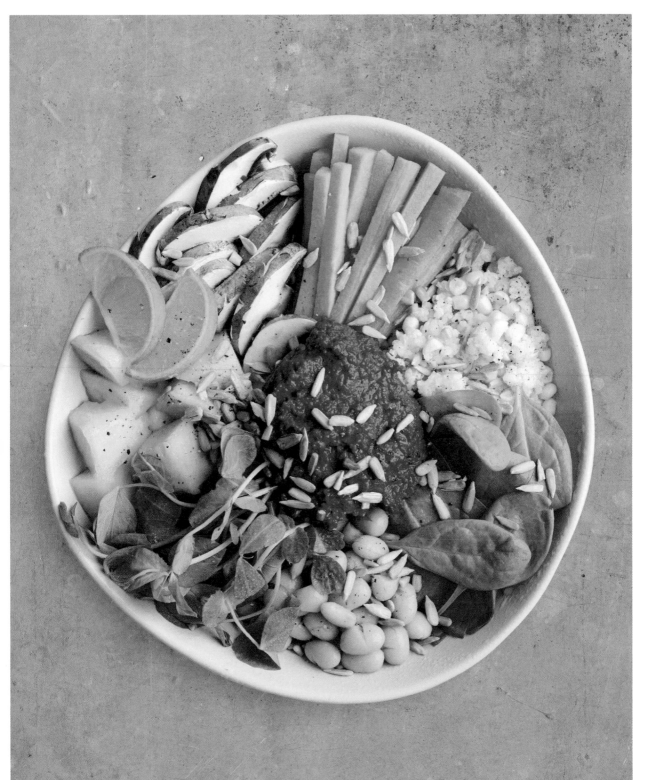

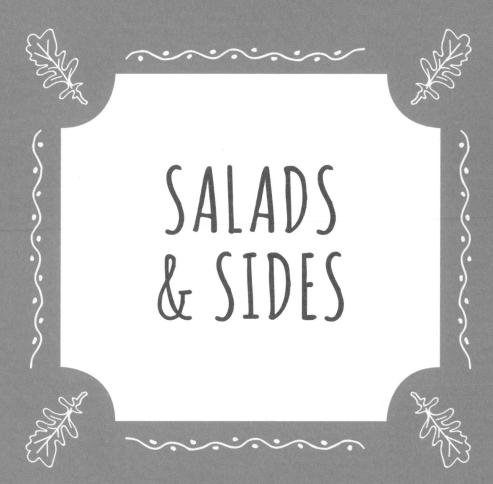

SALADS & SIDES

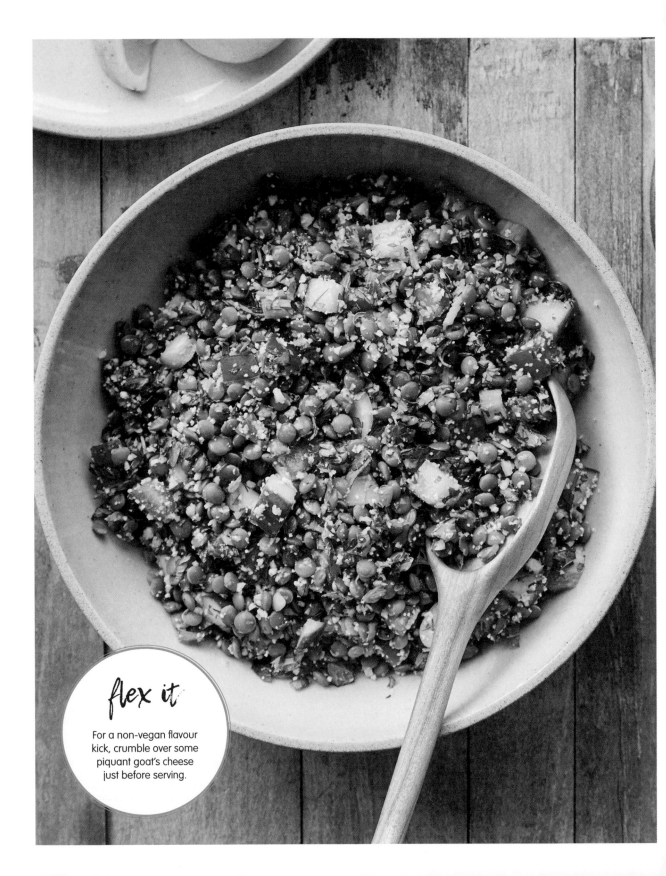

flex it

For a non-vegan flavour
kick, crumble over some
piquant goat's cheese
just before serving.

LENTIL & CAULIFLOWER TABBOULEH
with mint & lemon

SERVES 4
PREP 20 MINS

1 small **cauliflower head**
15g (½oz) chopped **flat-leaf parsley**
30g (1oz) chopped **curly parsley**
140g (5oz) **cucumber**, diced
175g (6oz) **tomato**, diced
1 small bunch **spring onions**, finely sliced
125g (4½oz) cooked **brown lentils**
15g (½oz) chopped **mint leaves**
zest and juice of 2 **lemons**
2 tbsp **olive oil**
salt and freshly ground **black pepper**

1 Remove the outer leaves from the cauliflower head and break it into florets. Place it in a food processor and pulse 6–7 times, until the cauliflower resembles rice or bulgur wheat.

2 In a large mixing bowl, combine the cauliflower, flat-leaf parsley, curly parsley, cucumber, tomato, spring onions, lentils, and mint. Add the lemon zest and juice and the olive oil and toss to combine. Season with salt and pepper to taste. Transfer to a serving dish and serve immediately.

VARIATION

For a zingy variation, add finely chopped red peppers, red onion, and chopped black olives into the mix in Step 2. Top with pomegranate seeds.

the good stuff

Using cauliflower as a grain is a great way to add nutrition and flavour to a dish. Cauliflower contains almost every vitamin you need, including vitamins C and B6, so is great for a plant-based diet.

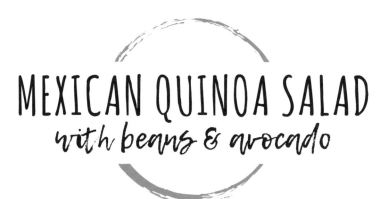

MEXICAN QUINOA SALAD
with beans & avocado

SERVES 2
PREP 15 MINS, plus cooling
COOK 20 MINS

50g (1¾oz) **quinoa**
400g (14oz) can **red kidney beans**, drained
50g (2oz) can **sweetcorn**, drained
½ **red onion**, finely chopped
1 **red pepper**, deseeded and finely chopped
4–6 slices pickled **jalapeño chillies**, finely chopped
1 **avocado**, pitted and cut into cubes
1 head of **romaine lettuce**
50g (1¾oz) plain **corn tortilla chips**, crumbled, plus extra to serve
1 **lemon** or **lime**, halved, to serve

1 Rinse the quinoa under running water, drain, and place in a lidded saucepan. Cover with 250ml (9fl oz) of water and bring to the boil.

2 Reduce the heat to a simmer, cover, and cook for 15–20 minutes or until almost all the liquid has been absorbed and the quinoa is fluffy. Remove from the heat, drain any remaining water, and set aside to cool.

3 Place the quinoa, kidney beans, sweetcorn, onion, pepper, and jalapeños in a large bowl. Mix until well combined. Then add the avocado and mix lightly to combine.

4 Roughly shred the lettuce and add to the bowl. Sprinkle the tortillas over the salad and toss lightly. Transfer to a serving platter or plate. Serve immediately with tortilla chips and lemons or limes to squeeze over.

the good stuff

Healthy eating guidelines tell us to eat a rainbow of foods for optimum nutrition – this dish will help you do just that with its colourful veg and high-protein beans and quinoa. Quinoa also has all the essential amino acids the body needs, so it is a must-have food on a vegan diet.

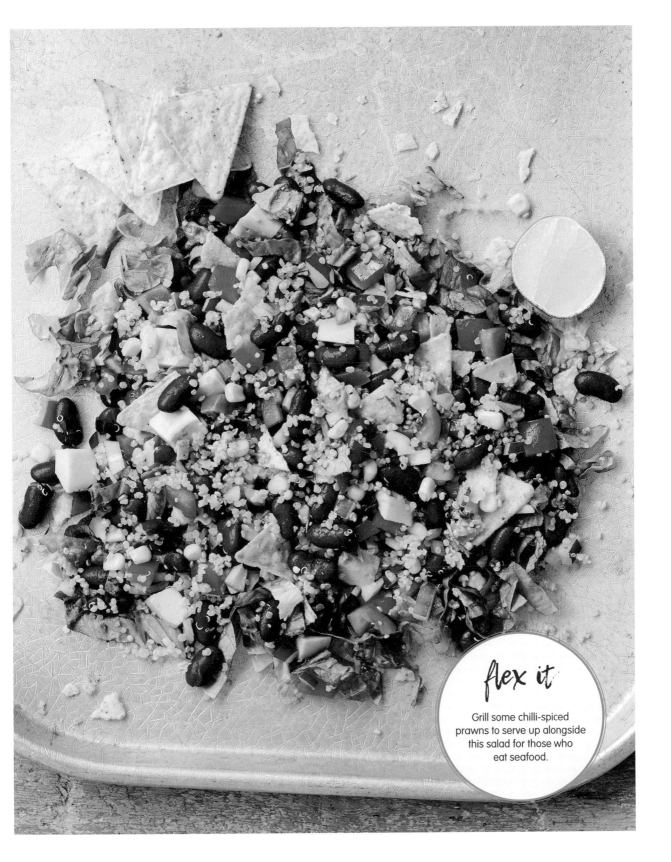

flex it

Grill some chilli-spiced prawns to serve up alongside this salad for those who eat seafood.

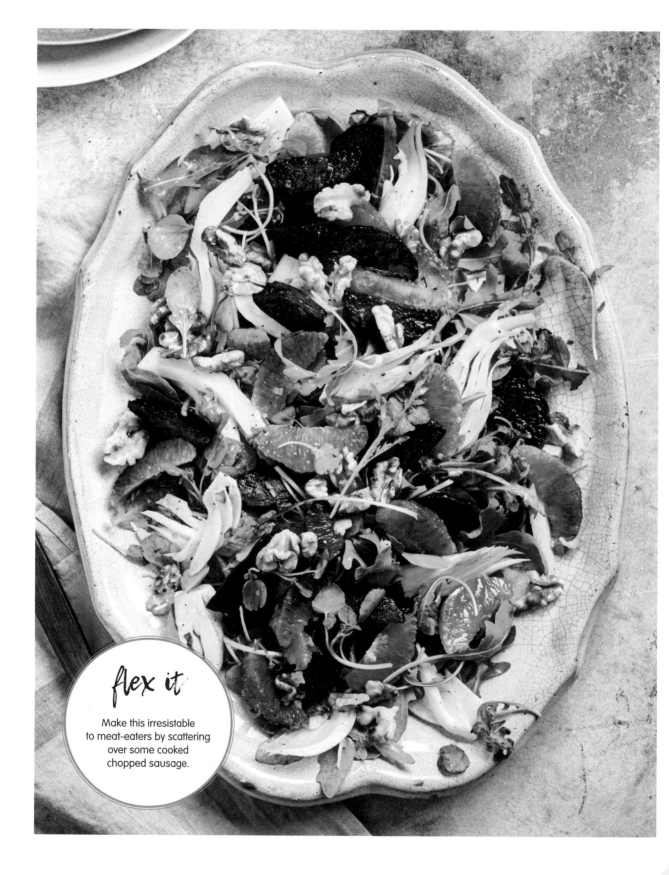

flex it

Make this irresistable
to meat-eaters by scattering
over some cooked
chopped sausage.

BLOOD ORANGE & BEETROOT SALAD
with fennel & walnuts

SERVES 4
PREP 20 MINS
COOK 30 MINS

2 medium-sized **beetroots**,
  peeled
1 tbsp **olive oil**
salt and freshly ground
  black pepper
30g (1oz) **walnuts**,
  roughly chopped
2 small **blood oranges**
1 small **fennel bulb**, trimmed
75g (2½oz) **watercress**, washed
  and dried
75g (2½oz) **baby rocket**,
  washed and dried

DRESSING
4 tbsp **extra virgin olive oil**
1 tsp **Dijon mustard**
salt and freshly ground
  black pepper

1 Preheat the oven to 200°C (400°F/Gas 6). Cut the beetroots into thin wedges, about 8 pieces per beetroot, and toss in the olive oil. Season well with salt and pepper, then roast for 30 minutes, turning once, until softened and charred at the edges. Set aside to cool.

2 Dry-fry the walnut pieces for 2–3 minutes over a medium heat, stirring constantly, until browned in places. Set aside to cool.

3 Prepare the oranges by peeling with a small, sharp knife, being careful to remove all the white pith. Use the knife to cut out each segment, leaving the dividing pith behind. Squeeze all the remaining juice out of the leftover orange "skeleton" into a bowl. Repeat with the second orange, setting the segments aside.

4 To make the dressing, add the olive oil, Dijon mustard, and seasoning to the extracted orange juice, and whisk well to combine. Slice the fennel very finely and toss it in the dressing immediately, to stop it discolouring.

5 Toss the prepared salad leaves with the fennel and dressing, then place on a large serving platter and top with the roasted beetroots, blood orange segments, and toasted walnuts. Serve immediately.

the good stuff

This sweet crunchy salad is high in potassium and vitamin C from the oranges, beetroot, fennel, and watercress, creating a super-charged meal that will keep your immune system healthy. Walnuts not only add flavour but are full of plant-based omega 3 fats.

ASIAN-STYLE SALAD
with sprouted mung beans & mint

SERVES 1
PREP 10 MINS

½ **courgette**, spiralized
8cm (3in) piece of **cucumber**, spiralized
30g (1oz) **sprouted mung beans**
30g (1oz) **pea shoots**
a few thin slices of **red onion**, to taste
2 tbsp roughly chopped **mint leaves**, plus extra to serve (optional)
1 tbsp roughly chopped **salted peanuts**

DRESSING
2 tbsp **rice wine vinegar**
2 tsp **sugar**
1 tsp **sesame oil**
½ tsp **soy sauce**, or **tamari**
¼ tsp finely grated **fresh root ginger**
¼ tsp finely grated **garlic**

1 To make the dressing, combine the vinegar, sugar, sesame oil, soy sauce, ginger, and garlic in a small bowl. Whisk until the sugar has dissolved.

2 Place the courgette, cucumber, sprouted mung beans, pea shoots, red onion, and mint in a serving bowl. Pour the dressing over the top and toss until the salad is well coated, piling the salad into the middle of the bowl.

3 Sprinkle with the chopped peanuts and a few extra mint leaves (if using) and serve immediately.

the good stuff

Sprouted mung beans may be little but they fill you up. They are also a great source of protein. Sprouted beans can carry harmful bacteria, so children, the elderly, pregnant women, and those with weakened immune systems should avoid eating them raw.

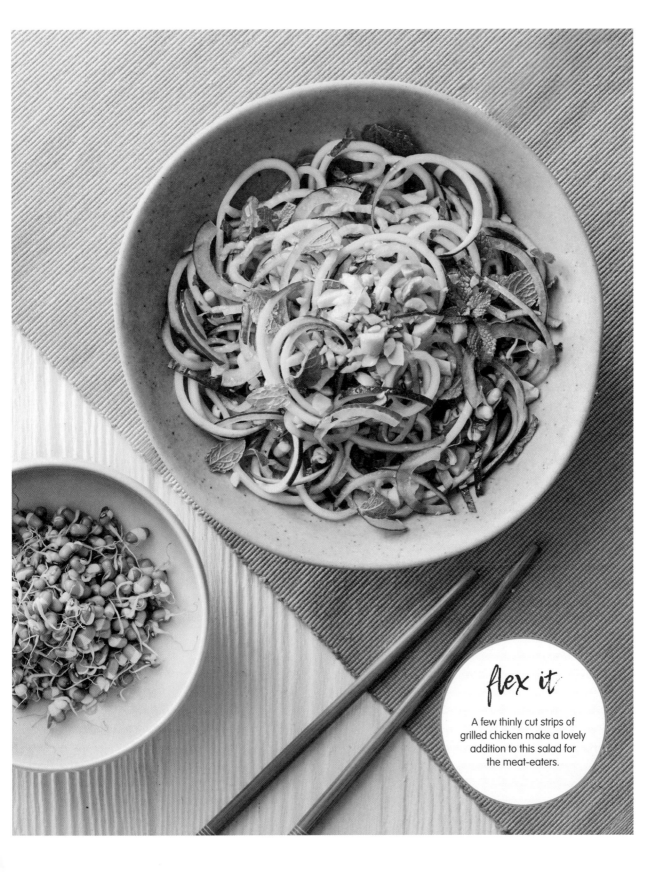

flex it

A few thinly cut strips of grilled chicken make a lovely addition to this salad for the meat-eaters.

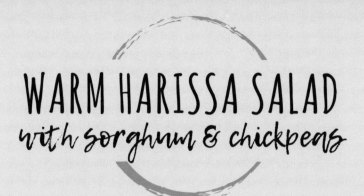

WARM HARISSA SALAD
with sorghum & chickpeas

SERVES 4
PREP 5 MINS
COOK 1 HR

200g (7oz) **sorghum**

2 **red peppers**, deseeded and
   cut into bite-sized pieces

2 **red onions**, diced

1 tbsp **light olive oil**

2 x 400g (14oz) can
   chickpeas, drained

1 tbsp **harissa paste**

juice of 1 **lemon**

salt and freshly ground
   black pepper

100g (3½oz) **rocket leaves**

4 tbsp roughly chopped
   flat-leaf parsley, to garnish

1 Rinse the sorghum under running water and place in a large,
lidded saucepan. Cover with water and bring to the boil. Reduce
the heat to a simmer and cook, covered, for 50–60 minutes, until
tender. Drain the sorghum and tip into a large bowl.

2 Meanwhile, preheat the oven to 200°C (400°F/Gas 6). Place the
red peppers and onions in a baking tray, drizzle with the olive oil
and toss to coat. Bake in the oven for 30–40 minutes, until softened.
Add the peppers and onions to the sorghum and mix well.

3 Add the chickpeas and harissa paste to the sorghum mixture.
Toss to combine, so the vegetables and chickpeas are evenly
coated. Pour over the lemon juice and season to taste. Divide the
rocket among 4 plates and top with the sorghum salad. Garnish
with parsley and serve immediately.

the good stuff

Sorghum is high in fibre and gluten-free
so it is a great alternative grain. It also contains
vitamins such as niacin, riboflavin, and thiamine.

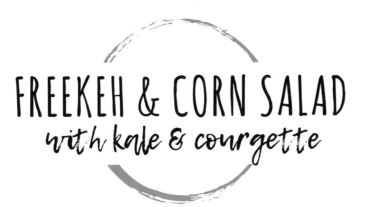

FREEKEH & CORN SALAD
with kale & courgette

SERVES 4–6
PREP 20 MINS, plus cooling
COOK 30 MINS

175g (6oz) **freekeh**
600ml (1 pint) **vegetable stock**
2 **corn on the cob**
1 tbsp **olive oil**
75g (2½oz) **almonds**,
   roughly chopped
30g (1oz) **sesame seeds**
10–12 **kale leaves**, ribs removed
   and finely chopped
425g (15oz) can **chickpeas**
4–6 **spring onions**, chopped
1 green **courgette**, diced
1 yellow **courgette**, diced

TAHINI DRESSING
3 tbsp **tahini**
1 **garlic clove**, pressed
2 tbsp **lemon juice**
1 tsp **low-sodium soy sauce**
1 tsp **toasted sesame oil**
salt and freshly ground
   black pepper

1 Rinse the freekeh under cold running water, drain well, and place in a lidded saucepan. Add the stock and bring to the boil. Then reduce the heat to a simmer, cover, and cook for about 20 minutes. Remove from the heat and leave to stand, covered, for 5 minutes. Uncover and leave to cool completely.

2 Bring a large pan of water to the boil. Add the corn and cook for 10 minutes or until the corn kernels are tender. Remove from the pan and rinse under cold running water. Remove the kernels from the cob by slicing down lengthways with a knife.

3 For the tahini dressing, place the tahini, garlic, lemon juice, soy sauce, and sesame oil in a small bowl. Add 2 tablespoons of water, and whisk until well combined. Taste, adjusting the seasoning if necessary, and set aside.

4 Heat the olive oil in a small non-stick frying pan over a low heat. Add the almonds and sesame seeds and toast for 2–3 minutes or until the almonds are lightly browned. Remove from the heat and leave to cool.

5 Place the kale in a large bowl and drizzle with some of the dressing. Toss well to coat. Then add the corn, almonds, sesame seeds, chickpeas, spring onions, and green and yellow courgettes. Drizzle over more of the seasoning and toss well to coat. Add the freekeh and the remaining seasoning and mix well to combine. Serve immediately.

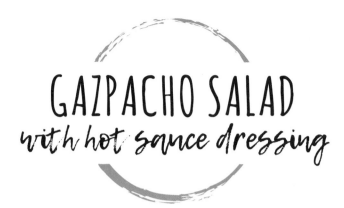

GAZPACHO SALAD
with hot sauce dressing

SERVES 2
PREP 15 MINS
COOK 15 MINS

2 **tomatoes**, quartered
1 tsp **olive oil**
pinch of **ground cinnamon**
pinch of **chilli flakes**
sea salt and freshly ground
   black pepper
85g (3oz) cooked **beetroot**,
   roughly chopped
70g (2¼oz) **cucumber**, sliced
¼ **red pepper**, roughly chopped
¼ **green pepper**, roughly chopped
1 **celery stick**, sliced
1 **garlic clove**, grated
1 **spring onion**, green part only,
   finely sliced
½ **avocado**
juice of 1 **lemon**
a few **basil leaves**

DRESSING
1 tsp **extra virgin olive oil**
a few drops of **hot sauce**

1 Preheat the oven to 200°C (400°F/Gas 6). Mix the tomatoes, olive oil, cinnamon, and chilli flakes in a roasting tin, and season with salt and pepper. Roast for 10–15 minutes, or until the tomatoes start to split. Set aside.

2 Mix the beetroot, cucumber, red pepper, green pepper, celery, garlic, and spring onion in a bowl.

3 Make the dressing by mixing the olive oil and hot sauce in a bowl, then toss it through the vegetables, add the roasted tomatoes, and toss again.

4 Chop the avocado roughly, then toss with the lemon juice to prevent discoloration.

5 Spoon the gazpacho salad into a serving bowl, then add the avocado and sprinkle over the basil leaves.

the good stuff

This is your 5-a-day in one bowl. Packed with goodness, the avocado provides a substantial amount of your daily monounsaturated fatty acids.

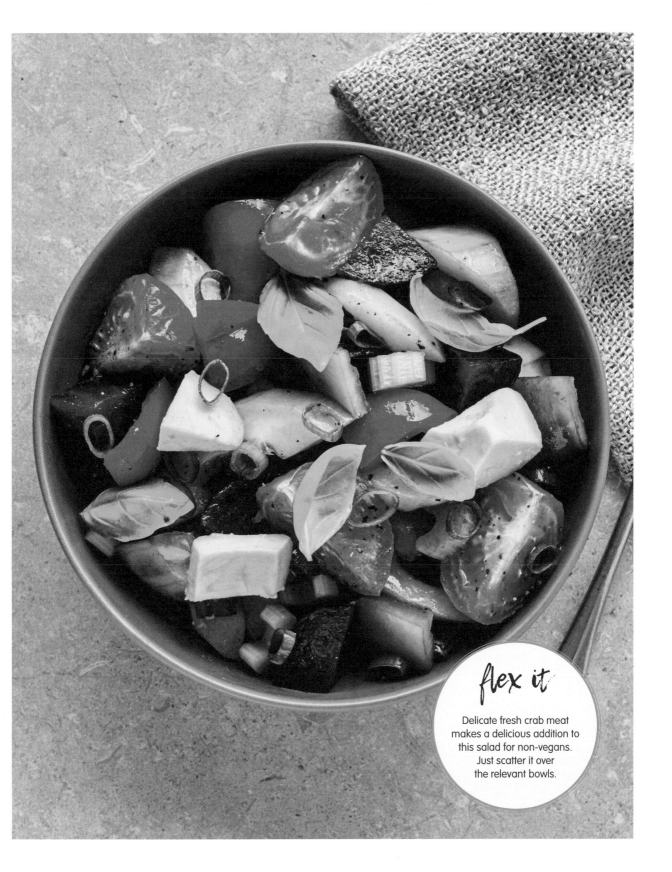

flex it

Delicate fresh crab meat makes a delicious addition to this salad for non-vegans. Just scatter it over the relevant bowls.

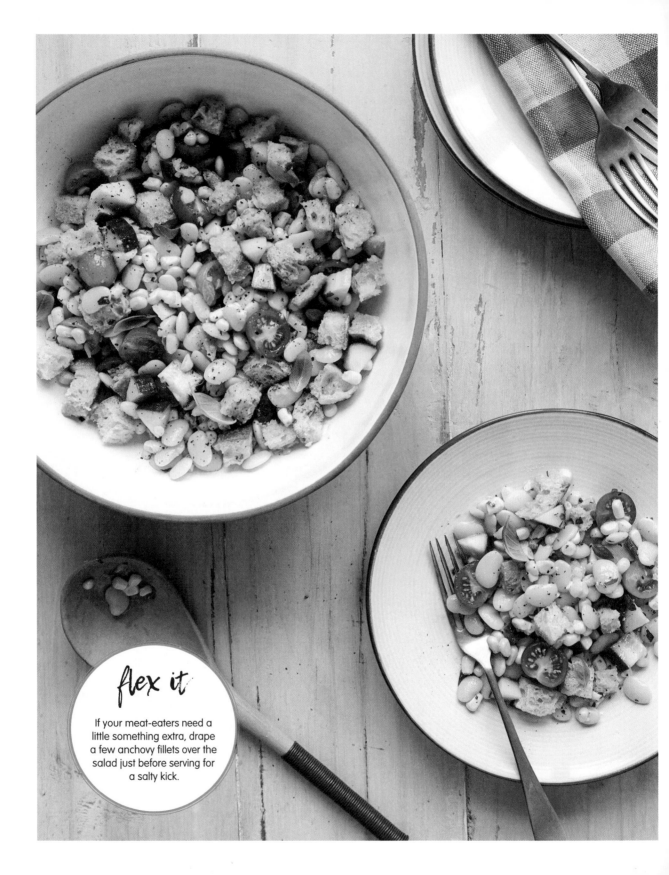

flex it

If your meat-eaters need a little something extra, drape a few anchovy fillets over the salad just before serving for a salty kick.

BUTTER BEAN PANZANELLA
with sourdough chunks

SERVES 6
PREP 25 MINS
COOK 15 MINS

1 small loaf **sourdough bread**
175g (6oz) **cherry tomatoes**, halved
225g (8oz) **cooked butter beans**
1 **cucumber**, diced
150g (5½oz) fresh
   sweetcorn kernels
salt and freshly ground
   black pepper

DRESSING
60ml (2fl oz) **red wine vinegar**
1 tbsp **Dijon mustard**
120ml (4fl oz) **olive oil**
2 **garlic cloves**, finely chopped
1 tsp chopped **oregano**
1 tsp chopped **basil leaves**

1 Preheat the oven to 170°C (325°F/Gas 3). Cut the bread into 1cm (½in) cubes. On a baking sheet, arrange the bread cubes in a single layer and bake for 15 minutes, or until toasted and light golden brown.

2 Meanwhile, to make the dressing, in a small bowl whisk together the vinegar and Dijon mustard. While whisking, drizzle in the olive oil and thoroughly combine. Stir in the garlic, oregano, and basil. Set aside.

3 To assemble, in a large salad bowl, add the tomatoes, butter beans, cucumber, and sweetcorn. Fold in the toasted bread, then drizzle the dressing over. Toss to coat. Season with salt and pepper to taste. Serve immediately.

the good stuff

Sourdough is more digestible than standard bread and the lactic acids make the nutrients in the flour easier for your body to absorb. Butter beans, with their high levels of B vitamins, are a must for the vegan pantry.

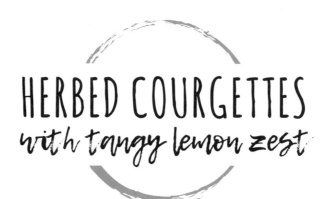

HERBED COURGETTES
with tangy lemon zest

SERVES 4
PREP 10 MINS
COOK 20 MINS

2 large **courgettes**

4 tbsp **plant-based mayonnaise**

250g (9oz) **panko breadcrumbs**

8 tbsp finely chopped fresh mixed herbs, such as **parsley**, **chives**, **chervil**, and/or **tarragon**

120ml (4fl oz) **extra virgin olive oil**

2 tsp **sea salt**

1 tsp freshly ground **black pepper**

2 tsp **lemon zest**

1 Preheat the oven to 200°C (400°F/Gas 6). Line a baking sheet with baking parchment.

2 Trim each courgette, cut into 5mm (¼in) slices. Blot dry with kitchen paper and brush both sides of each courgette slice with plant-based mayonnaise.

3 In a small, shallow bowl, combine the panko breadcrumbs, herbs, olive oil, salt, black pepper, and lemon zest.

4 Dredge each courgette slice in the panko mixture, coating both sides, and lay the slices on the prepared baking sheet.

5 Bake for 20 minutes, carefully turning with a spatula halfway through cooking, and serve immediately.

the good stuff

Fresh herbs are really good for you, as well as adding masses of flavour to plant-based dishes they contain flavonoids and have mild anti-inflammatory properties.

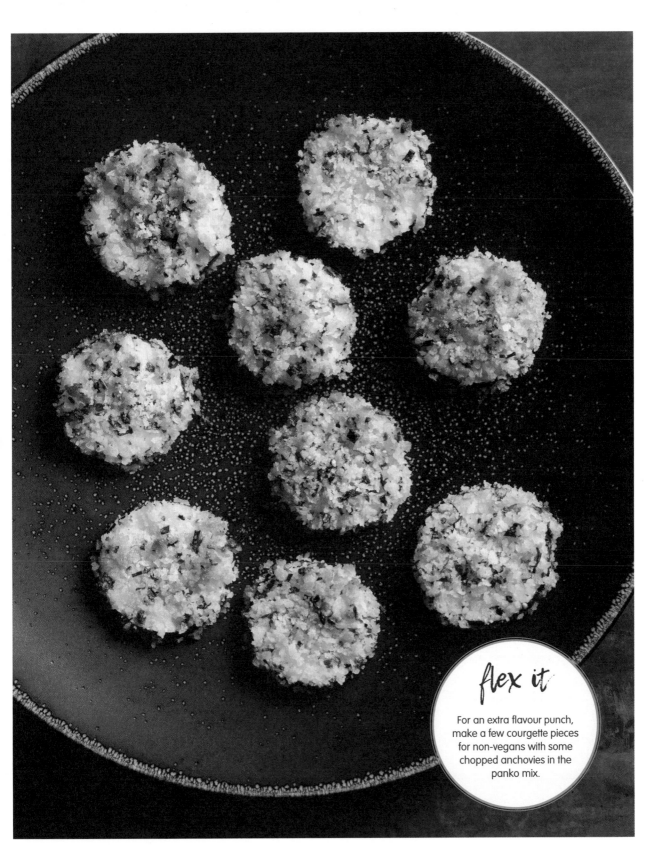

flex it

For an extra flavour punch,
make a few courgette pieces
for non-vegans with some
chopped anchovies in the
panko mix.

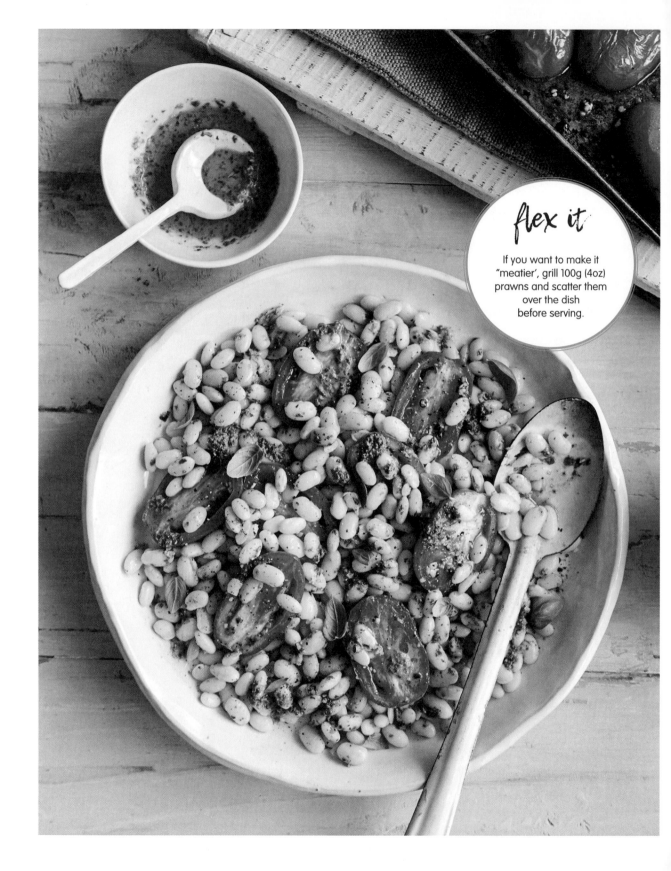

flex it

If you want to make it "meatier", grill 100g (4oz) prawns and scatter them over the dish before serving.

ROASTED TOMATOES & WHITE BEANS
with basil vinaigrette

SERVES 4
PREP 15 MINS
COOK 30 MINS, plus cooling

4 **plum tomatoes**
2 **garlic cloves**, finely chopped
1 tbsp **olive oil**
350g (12oz) cooked **cannellini**
　or **flageolet beans**

BASIL VINAIGRETTE
20g (¾oz) **basil leaves**,
　plus extra to garnish
60ml (2fl oz) **white wine** or
　Champagne vinegar
2 tbsp **olive oil**
salt and freshly ground
　black pepper

1 Preheat the oven to 200°C (400°F/Gas 6). Cut the tomatoes in half lengthways and toss with the garlic and the olive oil. Arrange on a baking tray and roast for 30 minutes. Let cool to room temperature.

2 Meanwhile, to make the basil vinaigrette, in a blender or food processor add the basil and vinegar. With the processor running on low, drizzle in the 2 tablespoons of olive oil until emulsified. Season with salt and pepper to taste.

3 In a mixing bowl, toss the beans with 2 tablespoons of dressing and spread on a serving plate. Arrange the roasted tomatoes on top. Season with salt and pepper. Garnish with any remaining dressing and basil leaves. Serve immediately.

the good stuff

As well as being packed with vitamins, tomatoes are also high in heart-healthy lycopene. Cooking tomatoes with a little oil makes it easier for your body to absorb this powerful nutrient.

GRILLED VEGETABLES
with garlic & parsley

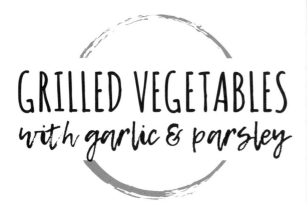

SERVES 4
PREP 20 MINS,
  plus marinating
COOK 10 MINS

2 **courgettes**, halved
  lengthways
1 large **red pepper,**
  quartered lengthways
  and deseeded
1 large **yellow pepper,**
  quartered lengthways
  and deseeded

1 large **aubergine**, sliced
1 **fennel bulb**, quartered
  lengthways
120ml (4fl oz) **olive oil,**
  plus extra for brushing
3 tbsp **balsamic vinegar**
2 **garlic cloves**, chopped
4 tbsp coarsely chopped
  flat-leaf parsley, plus
  extra to serve
salt and freshly ground
  black pepper

1 Arrange the vegetables, cut-side up, in a large
  non-metallic dish. Whisk together the olive oil,
vinegar, garlic and parsley, and season to taste
with salt and pepper. Spoon over the vegetables
and leave to marinate for at least 30 minutes.

2 Light the barbecue or preheat the grill on its
  highest setting. Grease the grill rack.

3 Lift the vegetables out of the marinade and
  place them on the barbecue or under the grill
for 3–5 minutes on each side, or until tender and
lightly charred, brushing with any extra marinade.
Serve sprinkled with parsley, with any remaining
marinade spooned over.

SPICED CHICKPEAS
with spinach

SERVES 4
PREP 10 MINS
COOK 10 MINS

3 tbsp **olive oil**
1 thick slice of **crusty
  white bread**, torn
  into chunks
750g (1lb 10oz) **spinach
  leaves**

240g (8½oz) **cooked
  chickpeas**
2 **garlic cloves**, finely
  chopped
salt and freshly ground
  black pepper
1 tsp **paprika**
1 tsp **ground cumin**
1 tbsp **sherry vinegar**

1 Heat 1 tablespoon of the olive oil in a frying pan
  and fry the bread, stirring, until crisp. Remove
from the pan, drain on kitchen paper, and reserve.

2 Rinse the spinach and shake off any excess
  water. Place it in a large saucepan and cook over
a low heat, tossing constantly so it does not stick
to the pan. When it has wilted, transfer the spinach
to a colander and squeeze out as much water as
possible by pressing it with a wooden spoon, then
place on a chopping board and chop coarsely.

3 Heat the remaining oil in the frying pan, add
  the spinach and allow it to warm through before
stirring in the chickpeas and garlic. Season to taste
with salt and pepper. Add the paprika and cumin,
then crumble in the reserved fried bread.

4 Add the vinegar and 2 tablespoons of water
  and allow to heat through for several minutes.
Divide among 4 small plates and serve immediately.

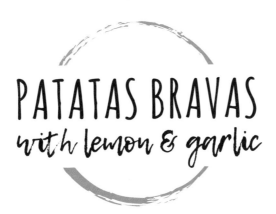

PATATAS BRAVAS
with lemon & garlic

SERVES 4
PREP 15 MINS
COOK 1 HR 10 MINS

6 tbsp **olive oil**
700g (1½lb) **white potatoes**,
   peeled and cut into 2cm
   (¾in) cubes
2 **onions**, finely chopped
1 tsp **dried chilli flakes**
2 tbsp **dry sherry (vegan)**
grated zest of 1 **lemon**
4 **garlic cloves**, grated or
   finely chopped
200g (7oz) can **chopped tomatoes**
small handful of **flat-leaf**
   parsley, chopped
salt and freshly ground
   black pepper

1 Preheat the oven to 200°C (400°F/Gas 6). Heat half the olive oil in a non-stick frying pan, add the potatoes, and cook over a low heat for 20 minutes, or until starting to brown, turning frequently. Add the onions and cook for a further 5 minutes.

2 Add the chilli, sherry, lemon zest, and garlic. Reduce for 2 minutes before adding the tomatoes and parsley. Season, combine well, and cook over a medium heat for 10 minutes, stirring occasionally.

3 Stir in the remaining oil, place all the ingredients in a shallow baking dish, and bake in the oven for 30 minutes, or until cooked. Serve hot with a selection of tapas dishes.

flex it

Keep die-hard meat-eaters happy by frying some slices of chorizo with a separate portion of potatoes, then add the flavourings and tomatoes.

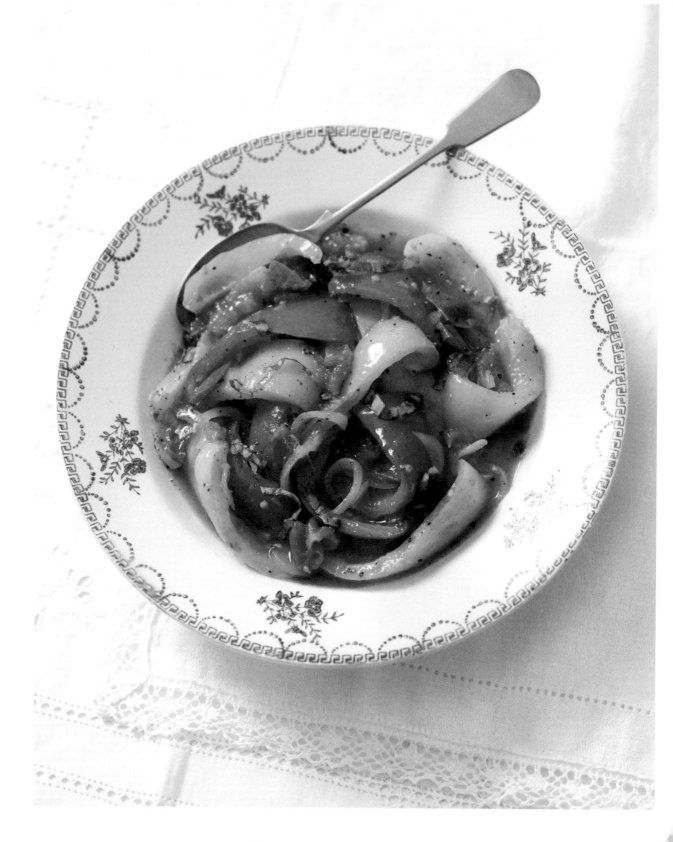

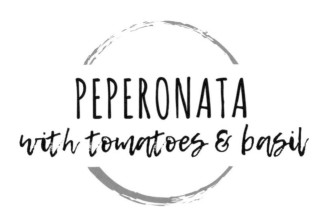

PEPERONATA
with tomatoes & basil

SERVES 4
PREP 10 MINS
COOK 40 MINS

2 tbsp **olive oil**

1 mild **onion**, finely sliced

1 **garlic clove**, crushed (optional)

2 large **red peppers** or 1 **red** and
  1 **yellow peppe**r, halved, cored,
  deseeded, and cut into strips

salt and freshly ground
  black pepper

4 ripe **tomatoes**, chopped

a few **basil leaves**, rolled
  and snipped

1 Pour the olive oil into a non-stick frying pan over a medium heat. Stir in the onion and cook for 5–8 minutes, until soft, stirring frequently. Add the garlic, if using, then stir in the peppers, season, and soften for 5 minutes, stirring often.

2 Add the tomatoes, stir well, and partially cover the pan. Cook for 20–30 minutes until just soft but not too mushy, stirring occasionally. Season to taste and stir in the basil. Serve warm or at room temperature.

VARIATION

For a tasty combination, add a chopped aubergine to the pan with the peppers. You could also stir in some cooked chopped potato.

the good stuff

Peppers add such a healthy kick to your meal as they are loaded with vitamins, especially C – just half a cup has almost double your daily needs.

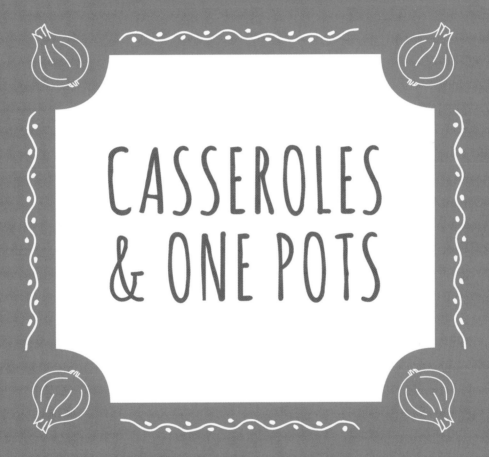

CASSEROLES & ONE POTS

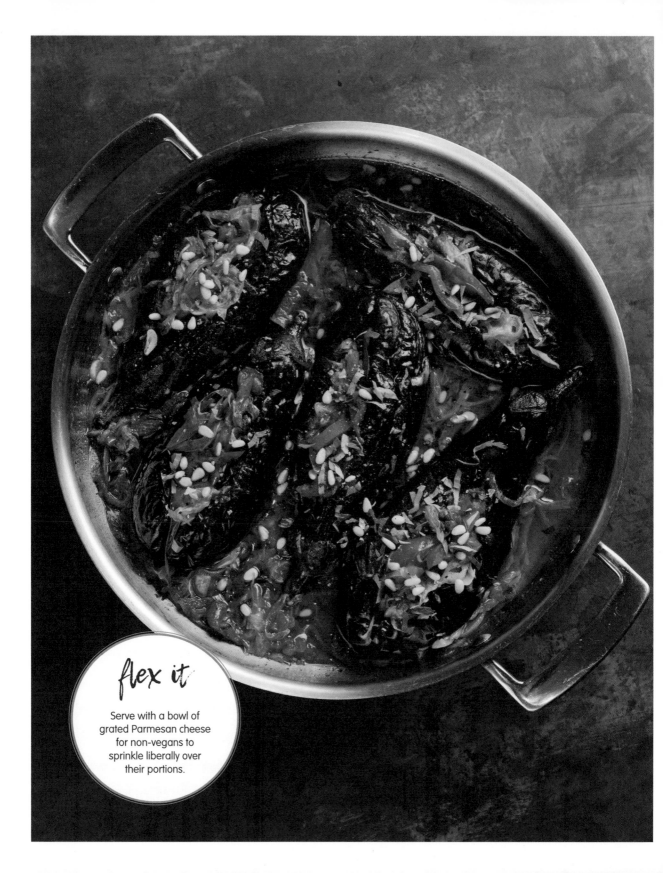

flex it

Serve with a bowl of
grated Parmesan cheese
for non-vegans to
sprinkle liberally over
their portions.

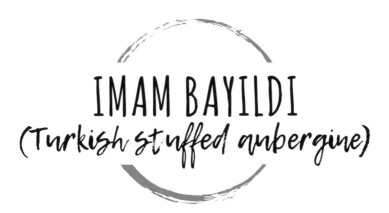

IMAM BAYILDI
(Turkish stuffed aubergine)

SERVES 6
PREP 15 MINS, plus soaking
COOK 1 HR 10 MINS

6 small **aubergines**
120ml (4fl oz) **extra virgin olive oil**,
 plus extra to taste
3 large **sweet onions**, halved and
 thinly sliced
6 ripe **plum tomatoes**, peeled,
 julienned, and juice reserved
6 **garlic cloves**, thinly sliced
4 tbsp **flat-leaf parsley**, finely
 chopped, plus extra to garnish
30g (1oz) **pine nuts**, toasted
 (optional)

1 Fill the kitchen sink or a large bowl with well-salted water. Cut a small slit in each aubergine, remove the stems (if desired), transfer them to the salt-water bath, and soak for 1 hour. Drain, squeeze gently, and pat dry.

2 Heat the olive oil in a wide, ovenproof frying pan or a cast-iron casserole dish with a lid over a medium heat. Add the onions and cook, stirring occasionally, for 5–10 minutes or until golden.

3 Add the aubergines, plum tomatoes, and garlic, reduce the heat to medium–low (adjust as needed), cover, and cook, stirring the onions once or twice without disturbing the aubergines, for 10 minutes.

4 Turn the aubergines and cook for another 10 minutes.

5 Preheat the oven to 190°C (375°F/Gas 5).

6 Remove the pan from the heat and gently stuff some onion–tomato mixture into each aubergine. Pour the reserved tomato juice over the aubergines, sprinkle with flat-leaf parsley, cover tightly with a lid or foil, and bake for 35–40 minutes.

7 Remove from the oven, and cool slightly before garnishing with toasted pine nuts (if using) and serving.

the good stuff

You can get your vital B vitamins from aubergines. Be sure to eat the skin, too, as this where all those health-boosting antioxidants are concentrated.

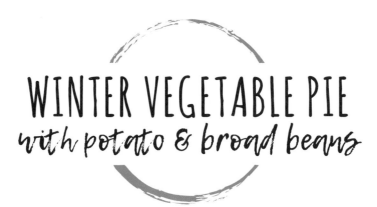

WINTER VEGETABLE PIE
with potato & broad beans

SERVES 6
PREP 15 MINS
COOK 45 MINS

4 tbsp **grapeseed oil**

3 tbsp **plain flour**

720ml (1 pint 4fl oz) **vegetable stock**

1 large **onion**, cut into small dice

4 large **celery sticks**, cut into small dice

3 **carrots**, cut into small dice

300g (10oz) **chestnut mushrooms**, quartered

3 **garlic cloves**, minced

4 large **red-skinned potatoes**, cut into small dice

1 **sweet potato**, cut into small dice

325g (11oz) **frozen broad beans**

1 **bay leaf**

1 tsp **dried thyme**

1 tsp **sea salt**, plus extra to taste

½ tsp freshly ground **black pepper**

1 sheet **vegan puff** or **shortcrust pastry**, thawed

1 Preheat the oven to 200°C (400°F/Gas 6). Heat 2 tablespoons of the grapeseed oil in a small saucepan over a medium heat. Whisk in the flour until smooth, and cook, stirring constantly, for about 2 minutes or until the flour is lightly golden and smells toasty.

2 Whisk in 480ml (16fl oz) of the vegetable stock, and simmer for 5 minutes. Remove from the heat, and set aside.

3 Heat the remaining oil in a wide frying pan over a medium–high heat. Add the onion, celery, carrots, mushrooms, and garlic, and cook, stirring frequently, for about 10 minutes, or until the vegetables are softened and beginning to colour.

4 Stir in the remaining stock, potatoes, sweet potatoes, broad beans, bay leaf, thyme, salt, and black pepper. Cover and cook, stirring once or twice and adding a bit of water if it seems dry, for 10 minutes.

5 Remove the bay leaf, stir in the reserved sauce, and pour the vegetable mixture into a 23 × 33cm (9 × 13in) baking dish.

6 Roll out the pastry on a floured surface to fit the top of the baking dish with an overhang of 1cm (½in). Prick all over with a fork, transfer it to the baking dish, and lay it gently over the vegetables. Tuck the overhanging edge down into the inside of the dish.

7 Bake for about 30 minutes or until the pastry is puffed and the filling is hot and bubbling. Serve immediately.

the good stuff

Comfort food can be nutritious – this pie is full of healthy root veg and broad beans, which are stuffed with protein and energy-giving folate as well as B vitamins.

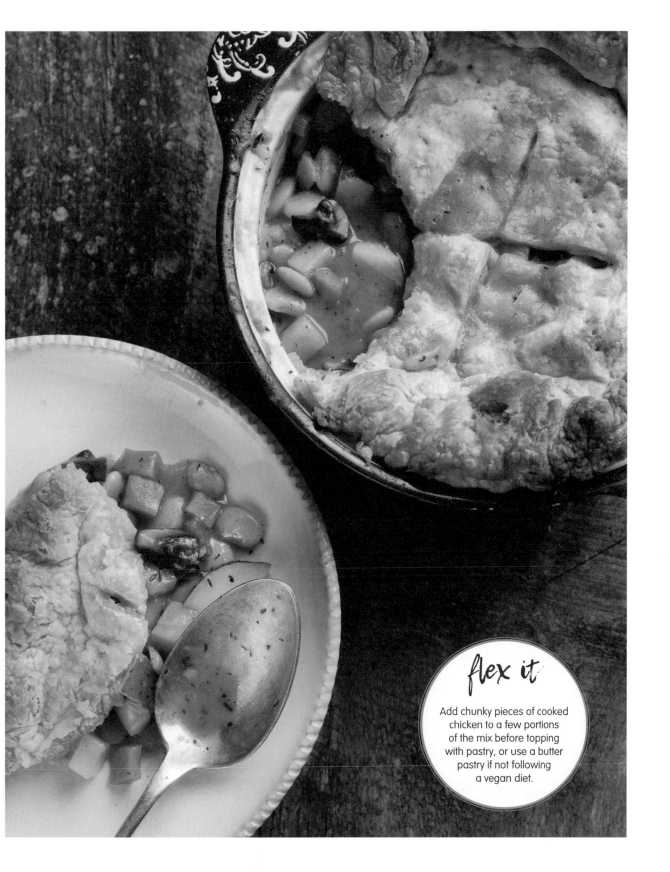

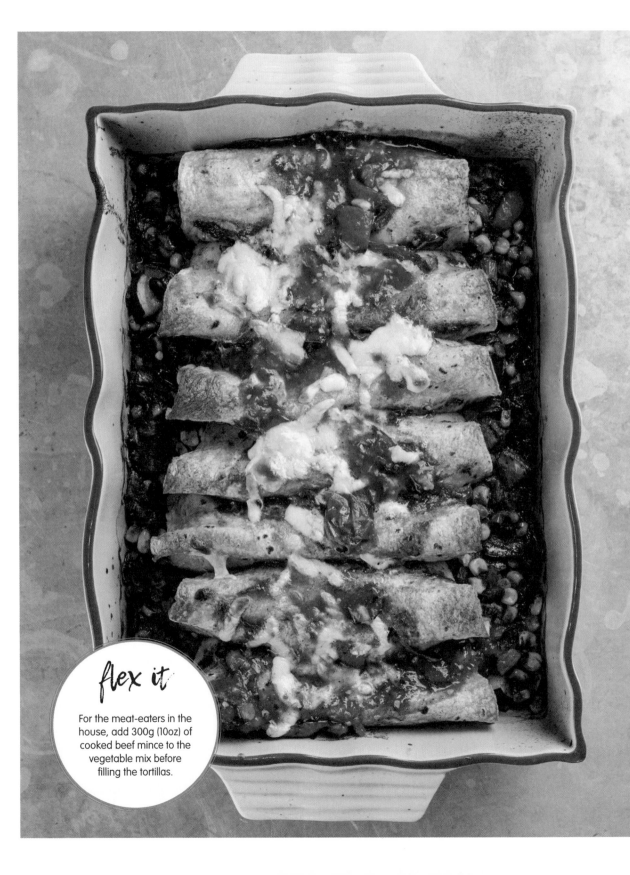

flex it

For the meat-eaters in the house, add 300g (10oz) of cooked beef mince to the vegetable mix before filling the tortillas.

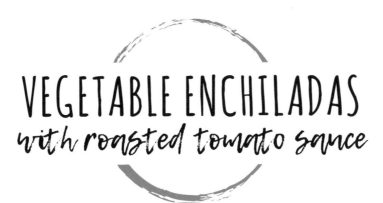

VEGETABLE ENCHILADAS
with roasted tomato sauce

SERVES 4
PREP 20 MINS
COOK 1 HR 40 MINS

4 tbsp **extra virgin olive oil**

550g (1¼lb) **small tomatoes**,
 such as Campari, cut in half

2 **red peppers**, deseeded,
 and cut into 2.5cm (1in) strips

1 tsp **sea salt**

½ tsp **dried oregano**

480ml (16fl oz) **vegetable stock**

3 tbsp **chilli powder**

1 large **onion**, finely chopped

2 **poblano chilli peppers**,
 deseeded and finely chopped

2 **garlic cloves**, finely chopped

2 large **courgettes**, cut into 1cm
 (½in) dice

450g (1lb) **roasted sweetcorn
 kernels**, or regular **frozen
 sweetcorn kernels**

1 x 400g (14oz) can **black beans**,
 rinsed and drained

2 tbsp finely chopped
 coriander leaves

16 x 15cm (6in) **tortillas**

60g (2oz) shredded **plant-based
 Cheddar–style cheese** (optional)

1 Preheat the oven to 190°C (375°F/Gas 5). Lightly coat
 a 23 × 33cm (9 × 13in) baking dish with a littleof the olive oil.
Place the tomatoes in the baking dish, and toss with 2 tablespoons
of the olive oil, red pepper strips, ½ teaspoon of the salt, and oregano.
Roast for 1 hour, stirring occasionally, and cool slightly.

2 Purée the tomato mixture, vegetable stock, and chilli powder
 in batches in a blender or a food processor. Set aside.

3 Heat the remaining oil in a wide frying pan over a medium–high
 heat. Add the onion and poblano chillies, and cook, stirring
occasionally, for 4–5 minutes, adjusting the heat as necessary. Add
the garlic, and stir for 1 minute. Add the courgettes, and cook for 4–5
minutes or until the vegetables are golden. Stir in the corn, and cook
for 1 or 2 minutes. Stir in the black beans, coriander, remaining salt,
and 120ml (4fl oz) of the reserved sauce. Remove from the heat.

4 Spread 120ml (4fl oz) of the sauce on the bottom of the dish.
 Spoon about one-twelfth of the filling into the centre of 1 tortilla,
filling it generously. Roll, and set in the dish. Repeat with the remaining
tortillas and filling, fitting tucking them in snugly. Pour over the
remaining sauce, lightly covering the enchiladas with the edges
exposed, and sprinkle with cheese (if using). Cover with foil, and bake
for about 40 minutes or until hot and bubbling. Serve immediately.

the good stuff

If you can handle the heat, hot chillies
are beneficial for health; the capsaicin
they contain is thought to have powerful
anti-cancer properties.

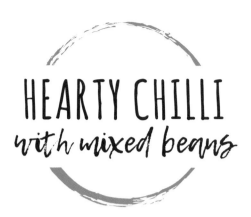

HEARTY CHILLI
with mixed beans

SERVES 6
PREP 10 MINS
COOK 1 HR

4 tbsp **extra virgin olive oil**

2 large **onions**, diced

4 **red peppers**, deseeded
and diced

2 **yellow peppers**, deseeded
and diced

300g (10oz) **chestnut mushrooms**,
thinly sliced

4 **garlic cloves**, finely chopped

1 tsp **sea salt**

2 tbsp **chilli powder**

1 tsp **ground cumin**

1 tsp **Anaheim chilli powder**

1 tsp **dried oregano**

1 tsp freshly ground **black pepper**

4 x 400g (14oz) can **chopped
tomatoes**, with juice

2 x 400g (14oz) can **kidney beans**,
rinsed and drained

2 x 400g (14oz) can **black beans**,
rinsed and drained

1 tbsp **habanero hot pepper
sauce**, plus extra to serve

**plant-based soured
cream** (optional), to serve

tortilla chips (optional), to serve

1 Heat the olive oil in a large, deep-sided pan or stockpot over
a medium heat. Add the onions, and red and yellow peppers,
and cook, stirring often, for 10 minutes.

2 Stir in the mushrooms, garlic, salt, chilli powder, cumin, Anaheim
chilli powder, oregano, and black pepper, and cook, stirring
frequently, for 10 minutes.

3 Add the chopped tomatoes, stir, and bring to a boil. Reduce the
heat to low or medium–low, and cook at a gently bubbling simmer,
uncovered, for about 30 minutes or until the peppers and onions are
very tender.

4 Stir in the kidney beans, black beans, and hot pepper sauce,
and cook for 5 minutes. Serve in big bowls with a spoonful
of plant-based soured cream (if using) and plenty of tortilla chips
(if using).

the good stuff

When eating a plant-based diet, try to introduce
beans daily, because they contain important
macro- and micronutrients, such as protein, iron,
zinc, folate, fibre, and potassium. They also
promote the growth of beneficial gut bacteria.

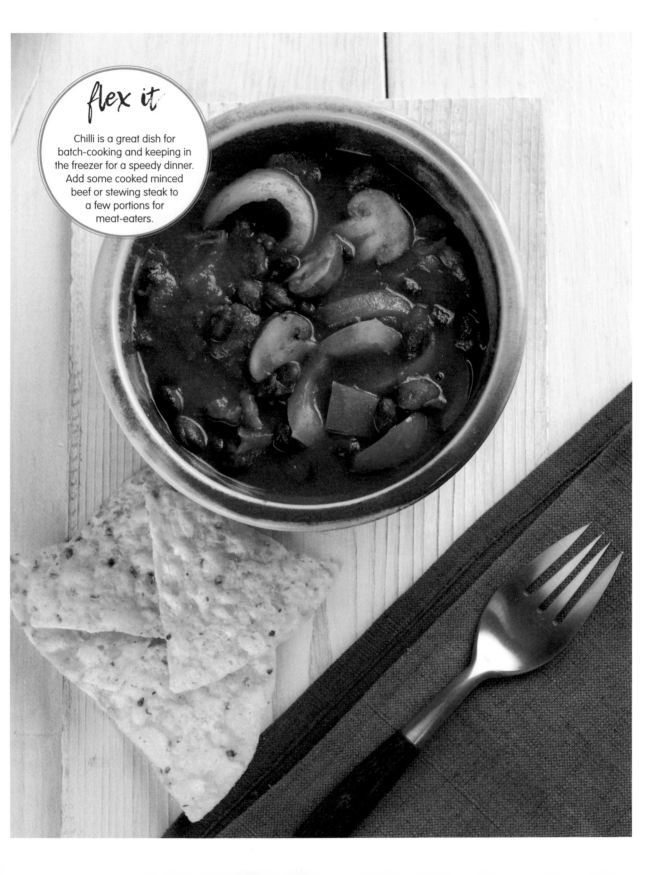

flex it

Chilli is a great dish for batch-cooking and keeping in the freezer for a speedy dinner. Add some cooked minced beef or stewing steak to a few portions for meat-eaters.

MOROCCAN SQUASH TAGINE
with pigeon peas

SERVES 6
PREP 45 MINS
COOK 40 MINS

1 tbsp **coconut oil**
1 **onion**, chopped
1 **carrot**, diced
2 **garlic cloves**, finely chopped
1 tsp grated **fresh root ginger**
1 tsp **smoked paprika**
1 **cinnamon stick**
¼ tsp **allspice**
½ tsp **ground coriander**
¼ tsp **ground cardamom**
2 tbsp **tomato purée**
475ml (16fl oz) **vegetable stock**
1 large **acorn** or **butternut squash**,
  peeled, deseeded, and diced,
  about 675g (1½lb)
325g (11oz) cooked **pigeon peas**
juice of 1 large **lemon**
75g (2½oz) **dates**, pitted
  and chopped
salt and freshly ground
  black pepper

1 In a tagine or large flameproof casserole, heat the coconut oil over a medium–low heat. Add the onion and carrot and cook for 2–3 minutes. Add the garlic and ginger and cook, uncovered, for an additional 1–2 minutes.

2 Add the paprika, cinnamon stick, allspice, ground coriander, and cardamom. Cook for 1 minute to warm the spices. Add the tomato purée and stock and stir to combine.

3 Stir in the squash and simmer, covered, for 15 minutes. Add the pigeon peas and cook for an additional 10 minutes, or until the squash is tender and the peas are warmed through. Stir in the lemon juice and dates. Season with salt and pepper to taste. Remove the cinnamon stick and serve immediately.

the good stuff

Dates contain B6 and magnesium and they make a great energy-boosting snack. However, they are also high in sugar, so only eat them in small amounts.

BLACK-EYED BEAN & COCONUT CASSEROLE
with garlic & ginger

SERVES 4
PREP 15 MINS
COOK 45 MINS

1 tbsp **olive oil**
1 **onion**, finely chopped
2 **garlic cloves**, finely chopped
5cm (2in) piece of **fresh root ginger**, peeled and finely chopped
1 **bay leaf**
1 tsp **coriander seeds**, crushed
2 x 400g (14oz) can **black-eyed beans**, drained and rinsed
400g (14oz) can **coconut milk**
600ml (1 pint) **vegetable stock**
3 **potatoes**, peeled and cut into bite-sized pieces
salt and freshly ground **black pepper**
200g (7oz) **basmati rice**

1 Heat the olive oil in a large pan, add the onion and cook until soft. Stir in the garlic, ginger, bay leaf, and coriander seeds, and cook for a couple of minutes, being careful not to burn the garlic.

2 Stir in the beans, then add the coconut milk and stock and bring to the boil. Reduce the heat and simmer, partially covered, for about 15 minutes. Add the potatoes and cook for a further 10 minutes or until they are done. If the casserole needs more liquid, top up with stock but don't let it become runny. Taste and season as needed and remove the bay leaf.

3 Meanwhile, put the rice in a large pan, cover with water and cook for 10–15 minutes, or according to the packet instructions. Once the rice is cooked, remove it from the heat, cover the pan, and leave it to steam for a few more minutes. Either add the rice to the casserole, or serve it separately.

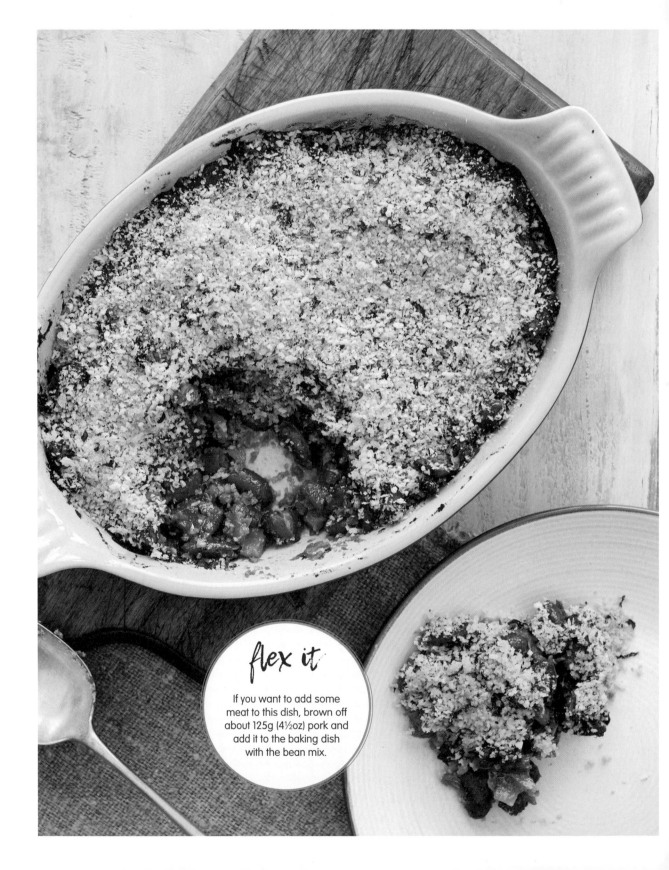

flex it

If you want to add some
meat to this dish, brown off
about 125g (4½oz) pork and
add it to the baking dish
with the bean mix.

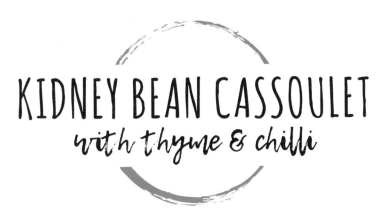

KIDNEY BEAN CASSOULET
with thyme & chilli

SERVES 4
PREP 20 MINS
COOK 45 MINS

2 tbsp **olive oil**
1 small **onion**, diced
1 **carrot**, diced
1 **celery stick**, diced
2 **garlic cloves**, finely chopped
3 sprigs of **thyme**
1 **bay leaf**
pinch of **crushed dried chillies**
300g (10oz) cooked **kidney beans**
175g (6oz) **passata**
180ml (6fl oz) **vegetable stock**
salt and freshly ground
   black pepper
50g (1¾oz) **panko breadcrumbs**
1 tbsp chopped **flat-leaf parsley**

1 Preheat the oven to 200°C (400°F/Gas 6). Lightly oil a 2-litre (3½-pint) baking dish.

2 In a stockpot or flameproof casserole, heat the olive oil over a medium–low heat. Add the onion, carrot, and celery, and cook for 2–3 minutes until soft. Add the garlic and cook for an additional minute.

3 Incorporate the thyme, bay leaf, chillies, kidney beans, passata, and stock. Simmer, covered, for 20 minutes.

4 Remove the bay leaf and thyme sprigs. In a blender or food processor, purée about 120ml (4fl oz) of the bean mixture until smooth. Return the puréed mixture to the pot and stir to combine. Season with salt and pepper to taste. Transfer the bean mixture to the baking dish.

5 To make the topping, in a small bowl combine the breadcrumbs and parsley. Top the dish evenly with the breadcrumb mixture. Bake for 20 minutes, or until golden brown. Serve immediately.

the good stuff

Kidney beans offer many of the key nutritional elements that are essential in a vegan diet; they are high in protein and fibre, and also provide potassium, phosphorus, iron, and thiamin.

POLENTA LASAGNE
with aubergine & roasted tomatoes

SERVES 6
PREP 45 MINS, plus chilling
COOK 1 HR 10 MINS

4 tbsp **extra virgin olive oil**
160g (5½oz) **coarse polenta**
  (not instant)
1½ tsp **sea salt**
1 large **aubergine**, cut into 2.5cm
  (1in) cubes
350g (12oz) **cherry tomatoes**,
  halved
3 **garlic cloves**, thinly sliced
360ml (12fl oz) homemade or
  bought **tomato sauce**
240ml (8fl oz) **dairy-free pesto**
6 large **basil leaves**, cut into
  thin ribbons
60g (2oz) **pine nuts**, toasted

the good stuff

Polenta is a cooked cornmeal that contains protein and fibre to help you feel full. The pine nuts are a good source of magnesium, which may help boost energy and fight fatigue.

1 Line a 23 × 23cm (9 × 9in) baking dish with baking parchment and brush it with a little olive oil. In a large saucepan over a high heat, bring 1.2 litres (2 pints) of water to the boil. Stirring constantly, add the polenta in a thin stream. Add ½ teaspoon of the salt, reduce the heat to medium, and stir until the polenta is fully cooked. (It will be creamy and smooth with no "bite"). Pour into the prepared baking dish and allow to cool. Cover and refrigerate for at least 2 hours or overnight until set.

2 Preheat the oven to 200°C (400°F/Gas 6). Sprinkle the aubergine cubes with ½ teaspoon of the salt and drain in a colander for 30 minutes. Rinse and gently squeeze out any water.

3 In a large baking tray, toss the aubergine and cherry tomatoes with garlic and 3 tablespoons of the olive oil. Spread evenly, and roast, stirring once or twice, for 30 minutes. Remove from the oven, and reduce the temperature to 190°C (375°F/Gas 5). When the polenta has set, carefully turn it out, cut into thirds, and slice each third horizontally into 3 equal pieces so you have 9 polenta "lasagne sheets". Handle carefully using a spatula – if they break, fit them together in the dish.

4 To assemble the lasagne, brush the baking dish with the remaining olive oil. Spread 120ml (4fl oz) of tomato sauce over the bottom and cover with 3 pieces of polenta. Top with half of the tomato–aubergine mixture and half of the pesto, followed by another polenta layer. Add another 120ml (4fl oz) of tomato sauce, the remaining aubergine–tomato mixture, and the remaining pesto. Top with the final layer of polenta and spread the remaining tomato sauce evenly on top. Cover and bake for about 40 minutes or until hot and bubbling.

5 Just before serving, sprinkle the basil and toasted pine nuts over the top of the lasagne. Serve hot.

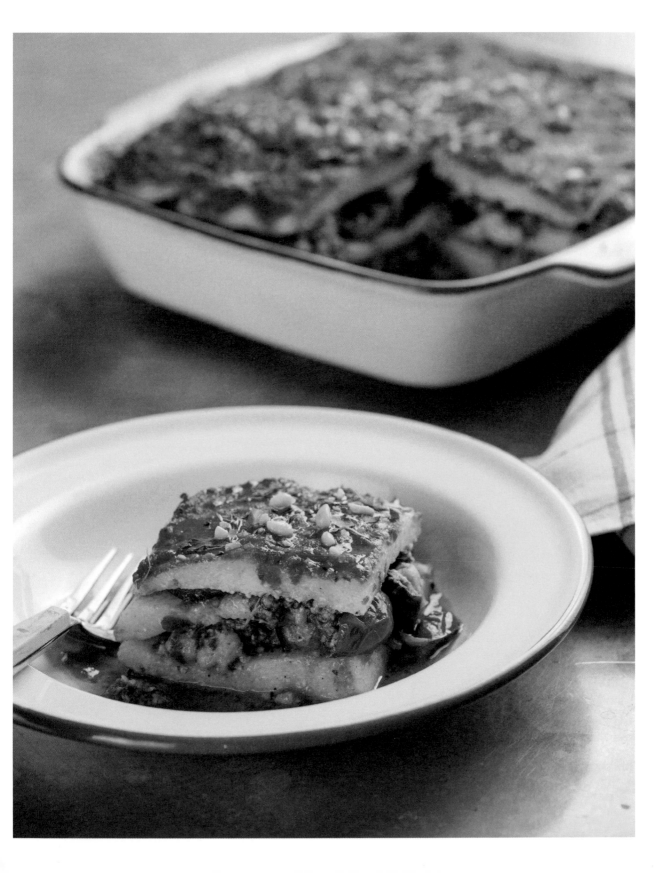

MUSHROOM LASAGNE
with shitake & porcini mushrooms

SERVES 8
PREP 30 MINS
COOK 1 HR 5 MINS

15g (½oz) **dried porcini mushrooms**
4 tbsp **extra virgin olive oil**
3 **garlic cloves**, minced
225g (8oz) **chestnut mushrooms**, thinly sliced
115g (4oz) **shiitake mushrooms**, stemmed and thinly sliced
1 tsp chopped **rosemary** or ½ tsp dried
1 tsp **sea salt**, or to taste
½ tsp **dried oregano**
½ tsp freshly ground **black pepper**, or to taste
4 tbsp **dry red wine**
960ml (1¾ pints) homemade or bought **tomato sauce**
9 ready-to-use **egg-free lasagne sheets**
480ml (16fl oz) **Cashew Ricotta (see p66)**

1 Preheat the oven to 190°C (375°F/Gas 5). Lightly coat a 23 × 33cm (9 × 13in) baking dish with cooking spray.

2 Place the porcini mushrooms in a small bowl, pour over 120ml (4fl oz) of boiling water, and soak for about 5 minutes or until softened. Lift the porcini from the water, agitating gently to release any soil. Reserve the soaking liquid. Chop the mushrooms and set aside.

3 Heat the olive oil in a large frying pan over a medium–high heat. Add the garlic and cook, stirring continuously, for 1 minute.

4 Add the porcini mushrooms, keeping the liquid, the mushrooms, rosemary, salt, oregano, and black pepper, and cook, stirring occasionally, for 10 minutes or until the mushrooms begin to brown.

5 Strain the mushroom liquid, leaving a few teaspoons behind to eliminate grit, and add to the mushrooms with the red wine, stirring vigorously to deglaze the pan. Stir until the liquid has evaporated, and set the mushrooms aside.

6 Spread 240ml (8fl oz) of tomato sauce evenly over the bottom of the baking dish, lay 3 sheets of lasagne over the sauce, spoon half of the mushroom mixture and half of the Cashew Ricotta evenly over the lasagne sheets. Pour 180ml (6fl oz) of tomato sauce over the Cashew Ricotta, layer a further 3 lasagne sheets, add the remaining mushrooms and Cashew Ricotta, followed by another 180ml (6fl oz) of tomato sauce. Finish with 3 lasagne sheets and another 180ml (6fl oz) of tomato sauce. Cover with foil, folding back a corner slightly to allow steam to escape. Reserve the remaining 120ml (4fl oz) of sauce to serve.

7 Bake for 50 minutes or until bubbling. Set aside for 5–10 minutes before cutting. Reheat the remaining sauce before serving.

SQUASH & ONION BAKE
with nutmeg & rosemary

SERVES 4
PREP 15 MINS
COOK 45 MINS

4 tbsp **extra virgin olive oil**
2 large **sweet onions**, thinly sliced
   into rings
2 **garlic cloves**, finely chopped
2 **courgettes**, thinly sliced
2 **yellow squash**, thinly sliced
1 tsp **sea salt**
¼ tsp freshly ground **black pepper**
2 tbsp **plain flour**
360ml (12fl oz) **non-dairy milk**,
   such as **rice** or **soya milk**
¼ tsp **ground nutmeg**
½ tsp finely chopped **rosemary**
115g (4oz) **panko breadcrumbs**
2 tbsp finely chopped **chives**
1 tsp **dried thyme**

flex it

For a meaty version, cook
300g (10oz) of minced beef
or pork with the onions, and
assemble and bake as
per the recipe.

1 Preheat the oven to 180°C (350°F/Gas 4). Lightly grease a 20 x 20cm (8 × 8in) square baking dish.

2 Heat 2 tablespoons of the olive oil in a wide frying pan over a medium–high heat. Add the onions and cook, stirring, for 5 minutes or until softened.

3 Add the garlic and stir for 1 minute. Remove the onions and garlic from the pan and keep warm.

4 Add 1 tablespoon of the olive oil, courgettes, and yellow squash, and season with salt and black pepper. Increase the heat to high and cook, stirring every minute or so, for 5 minutes or until the vegetables begin to turn golden.

5 Sprinkle with the flour, reduce the heat to medium, and stir for 1 minute to combine well. Return the onion mixture to the pan.

6 Stir in the non-dairy milk, nutmeg, and rosemary. Bring to the boil, and cook for about 2 minutes or until thickened.

7 In a small bowl, combine the panko breadcrumbs, chives, thyme, and the remaining olive oil.

8 Gently spread the squash mixture in the baking dish, and sprinkle evenly with the breadcrumbs. Bake, uncovered, for 30 minutes. Serve immediately.

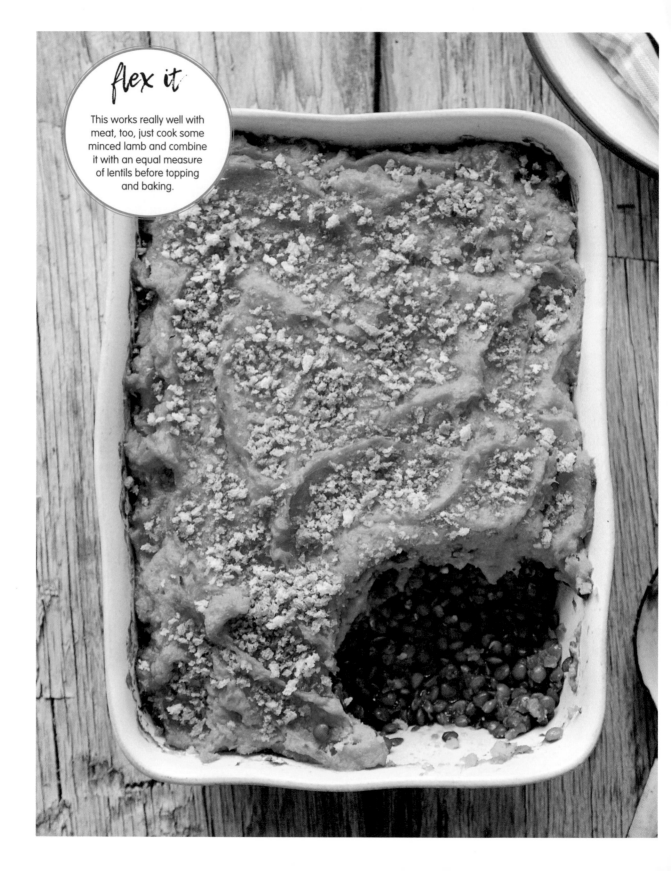

SPICED SWEET POTATO SHEPHERD'S PIE
with cumin & turmeric

SERVES 6
PREP 35 MINS
COOK 50 MINS

3 **sweet potatoes**, peeled
  and diced
75ml (2½fl oz) **plant-based cream**
salt and freshly ground
  black pepper
1 tbsp **olive oil**
1 **onion**, chopped
1 **garlic clove**, finely chopped
500g (1lb 2oz) cooked
  brown lentils
1 tbsp **ground cumin**
1 tbsp **garam masala**
2 tsp **curry powder**
1 tsp **ground turmeric**
400ml (14fl oz) **vegetable stock**
15g (½oz) chopped
  coriander leaves
45g (1½oz) **panko breadcrumbs**

1 Preheat the oven to 190°C (375°F/Gas 5). In a large saucepan, bring 1.5 litres (2½ pints) of water to the boil. Cook the potatoes for 15–20 minutes until tender. Drain thoroughly and transfer to a large mixing bowl. With a potato masher, mash the potatoes and plant-based cream until smooth. Season with salt and pepper to taste.

2 Meanwhile, in a large frying pan warm the olive oil over a medium heat. Add the onion and cook for 2 minutes, or until soft. Add the garlic and cook for an additional minute.

3 Add the lentils, cumin, garam masala, curry powder, and turmeric. Stir to combine and cook for 1–2 minutes to warm the spices. Add the stock and cook for 5 minutes. Stir in the chopped coriander.

4 Pour the lentil mixture evenly into a 23 × 30cm (9 x 12in) glass or ceramic baking dish. Top with the mashed sweet potato. Bake for 15 minutes. Sprinkle evenly with the breadcrumbs and bake for another 10 minutes, or until lightly browned. Cool for 10 minutes before serving.

the good stuff

Everyone can benefit from including nutritional lentils in their diet – they will give you slow, steady energy, and are also a quick-cooking and tasty plant-based protein.

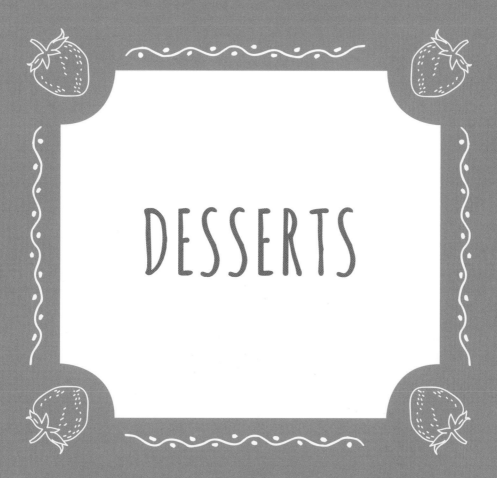

DESSERTS

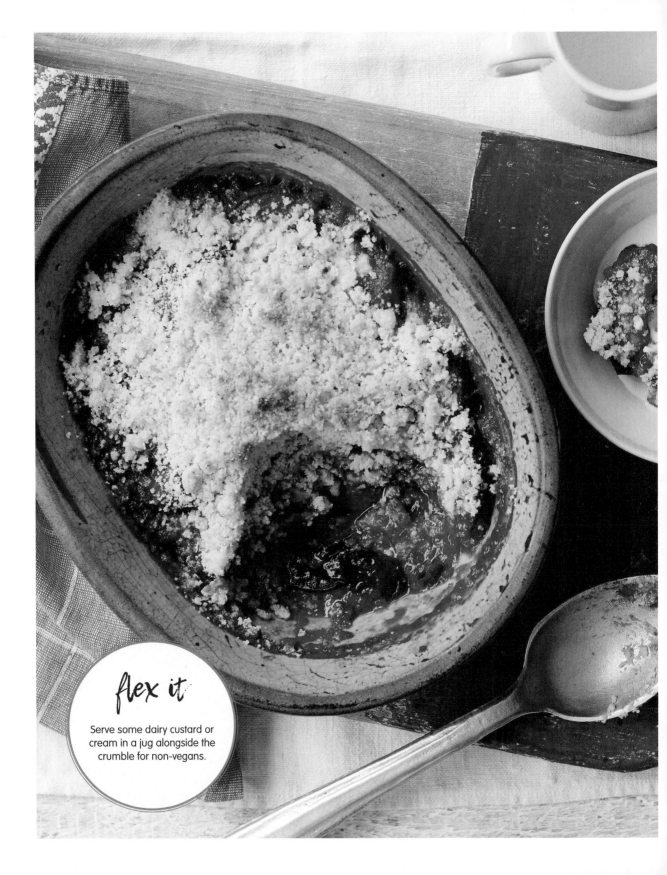

flex it

Serve some dairy custard or cream in a jug alongside the crumble for non-vegans.

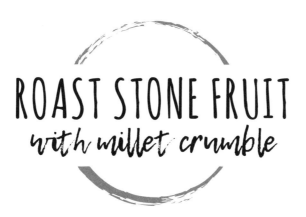

ROAST STONE FRUIT
with millet crumble

SERVES 4
PREP 15 MINS, plus cooling
COOK 1 HR

FRUIT FILLING
800g (1¾lb) **mixed fruit**, such as
  peaches, **nectarines**, and **plums**,
  stoned and roughly chopped
1 tbsp **coconut oil**,
  at room temperature

CRUMBLE TOPPING
85g (3oz) **millet flakes**
85g (3oz) **ground almonds**
50g (1¾oz) **coconut oil**,
  chilled and diced
60g (2oz) **unrefined caster sugar**

plant-based cream, to serve

1 Preheat the oven to 200°C (400°F/Gas 6). For the filling, place the
fruit in a roasting tray, drizzle over the coconut oil, and toss to coat.
Roast in the oven for 20–30 minutes, until tender but still holding their
shape. Remove from the oven and leave to cool for at least 10 minutes.

2 For the crumble topping, place the millet flakes and almonds in a
bowl and mix well to combine. Rub in the oil and mix well until the
mixture resembles rough breadcrumbs. Add the sugar and gently mix
to combine.

3 Place the cooled fruit mixture in a 20 x 25cm (8 x 10in) shallow
baking dish and spread it out in an even layer. Sprinkle the topping
evenly over the fruit. Place in the oven and bake for 20–30 minutes,
until the topping is golden brown. Remove from the heat and
serve warm with some plant-based cream.

the good stuff

Stone fruits are low in saturated fat and
cholesterol and are a good source of fibre.
Topped with healthy millet flakes that are
full of magnesium and calcium, this is
a good-for-you dessert.

ADZUKI BEAN CHOCOLATE PUDDING
with fresh raspberries

SERVES 6
PREP 10 MINS, plus cooling
  and chilling
COOK 10 MINS

3 tbsp **cornflour**
200g (7oz) cooked **adzuki beans**
240ml (8fl oz) **unsweetened
  almond milk**
2 tsp **vanilla bean paste**
60ml (2fl oz) **agave nectar**
45g (1½oz) **vegan unsweetened
  cocoa powder**
6 **raspberries**, to decorate

1 In a small bowl, whisk together the cornflour and 2 tablespoons of water. Set aside.

2 In a blender, purée the adzuki beans with 80ml (2¾fl oz) of water and 120ml (4fl oz) of the almond milk until smooth.

3 In a small saucepan, whisk together the remaining 120ml (4fl oz) of almond milk, the vanilla bean paste, agave, cocoa powder, and puréed adzuki beans until completely smooth.

4 Heat the almond milk mixture over a low heat for 8–10 minutes until the mixture reaches a low simmer, stirring occasionally to avoid lumps. Remove from the heat and let sit at room temperature for 10 minutes.

5 Divide evenly among 6 serving cups, cover, and refrigerate overnight to set. Top each with a raspberry before serving.

the good stuff

This recipe is a clever way to make a chocolate pudding healthy. To really boost the nutritional benefits, use an almond milk that is fortified with calcium.

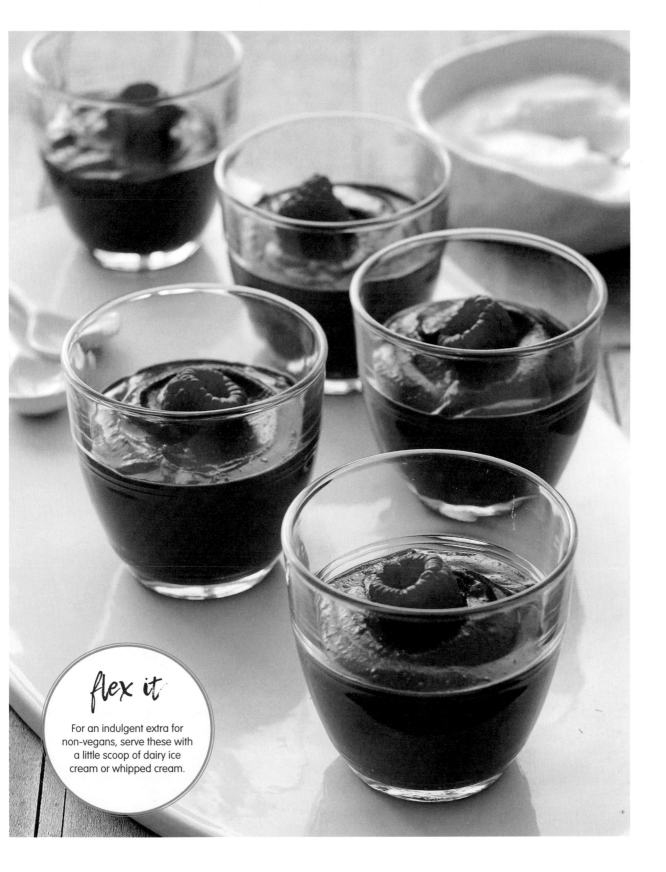

flex it

For an indulgent extra for non-vegans, serve these with a little scoop of dairy ice cream or whipped cream.

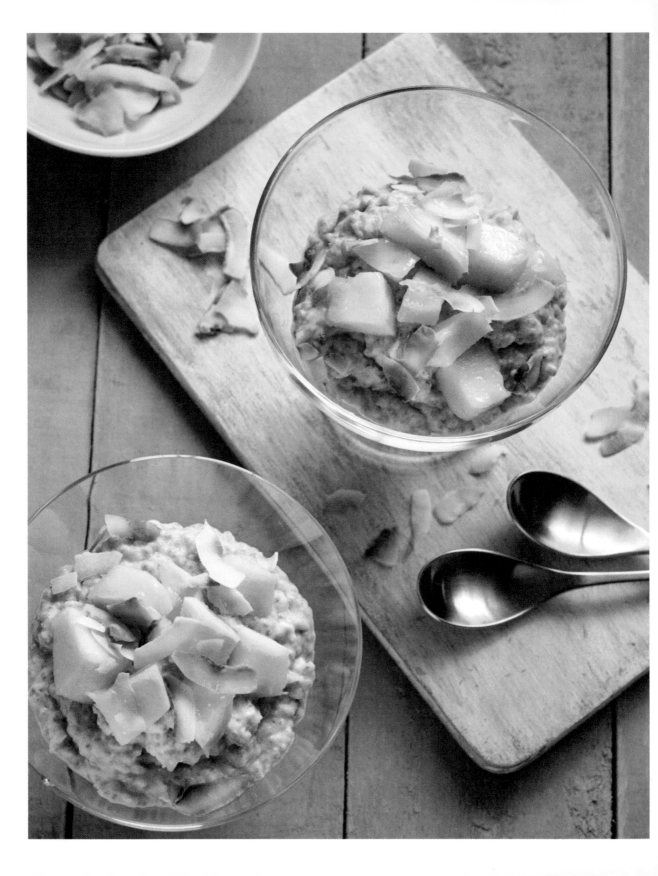

COCONUT & MANGO CHIA PUDDING
with toasted coconut flakes

SERVES 4
PREP 10 MINS, plus chilling

flesh of 1 large **mango**, about
   115g (4oz), chopped, plus extra
   to serve
300ml (10fl oz) **reduced-fat
   coconut milk**
30g (1oz) **chia seeds**
1 tbsp **maple syrup**
toasted coconut flakes,
   to serve (optional)

1 Place the mango and coconut milk in a food processor or blender and blend until smooth.

2 Add the chia seeds and maple syrup and blend briefly to combine. Place the mixture in a bowl, cover, and refrigerate overnight.

3 If the pudding is too thick the next day, loosen it with a little coconut milk until it reaches your desired consistency.

4 To serve, top the pudding with chopped fresh mango and toasted coconut flakes.

the good stuff

Mango not only boosts your vitamin C intake, but also helps to keep your eyes healthy, thanks to the antioxidant zeaxanthan. As an added nutritional burst, fibre-packed chia seeds are rich in essential magnesium.

FLOURLESS BLACK BEAN BROWNIES
with vanilla & orange

MAKES 12
PREP 15 MINS
COOK 35 MINS, plus cooling

400g (14oz) can **black beans**,
    drained, 9 tbsp of the liquid
    (aquafaba) reserved
120ml (4fl oz) **agave nectar**
60g (2oz) **coconut oil**
1 tsp **vanilla extract**
zest of 1 **orange**
¼ tsp **salt**
½ tsp **baking powder**
75g (2½oz) **caster sugar**
45g (1½oz) **unsweetened**
    cocoa powder
85g (3oz) **vegan dark**
    chocolate chips

1 Preheat the oven to 180°C (350°F/Gas 4). Lightly oil a 28 x 18cm (11 x 7in) metal baking tin. In a food processor, combine the black beans, agave, coconut oil, vanilla extract, and orange zest until smooth.

2 In a large mixing bowl, combine the salt, baking powder, sugar, and cocoa powder. Incorporate the black bean mixture and aquafaba until well mixed.

3 Gently fold in the chocolate chips, being careful not to overwork the mixture.

4 Pour the mixture into the baking tin. Bake for 30–35 minutes, until the brownies pull away from the edge and a skewer inserted into the centre comes out clean. Leave to cool for 15–20 minutes before cutting and serving.

the good stuff

Nice but not so naughty – the low glycaemic load in beans will help to keep your sugar levels stable so you won't peak and trough like you would eating regular brownies.

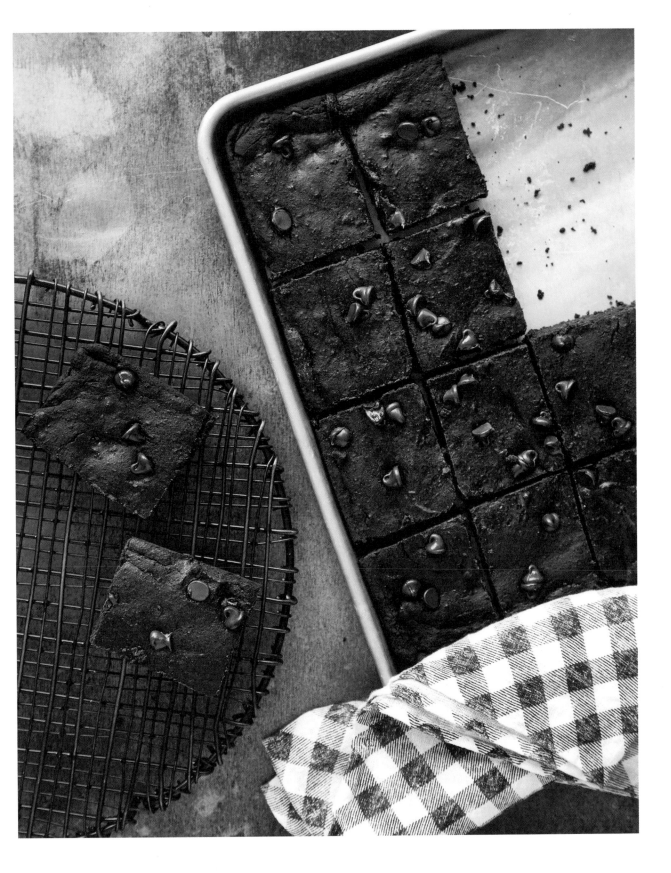

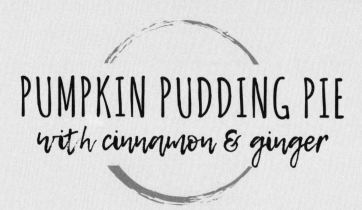

PUMPKIN PUDDING PIE
with cinnamon & ginger

SERVES 10
PREP 10 MINS, plus cooling
   and chilling
COOK 30 MINS

300g (10oz) **vegan gingernut**
   biscuits
4 tbsp melted **plant-based butter**
   or **coconut oil**
2 tsp **sea salt**
4 tbsp **instant tapioca**, such
   as Minute Tapioca
1 tsp **ground cinnamon**
½ tsp **ground ginger**
125g (4½oz) **brown sugar**
240ml (8fl oz) **coconut**
   milk creamer
240ml (8fl oz) **unsweetened**
   almond milk
1 tbsp **maple syrup**
1 tsp **vanilla extract**
4 tbsp **cornflour**
425g (15oz) can **pumpkin purée**

1 Preheat the oven to 180°C (350°F/Gas 4). In a food processor fitted with a metal blade, process the gingernuts, butter, and 1 teaspoon of the salt until the mixture resembles coarse crumbs. Press this into a deep 25cm (10in) pie dish, place the dish on a baking sheet, and bake for 20 minutes. Remove from the oven, and set aside to cool.

2 Meanwhile, in a medium saucepan, whisk together the instant tapioca, cinnamon, ginger, brown sugar, and remaining salt. Place the pan on the hob, set the heat to low, and slowly whisk in the coconut milk coffee creamer, half of the almond milk, maple syrup, and vanilla extract. Increase the heat to medium and bring to the boil.

3 In a small bowl, whisk together the cornflour and remaining almond milk. Whisk this mixture into the tapioca mixture and continue whisking slowly for about 3 minutes or until the mixture has thickened.

4 Whisk in the pumpkin purée, remove from the heat, and cool for 10 minutes.

5 Pour the pumpkin pudding into the baked biscuit crust, spreading with a spatula to smooth the top. Cool for 10 minutes, cover with cling film (or invert a large glass bowl over the top), and refrigerate overnight. Store any leftover pie in the fridge for up to 2 days.

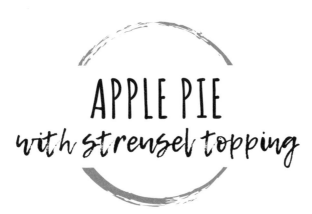

APPLE PIE
with streusel topping

SERVES 8
PREP 25 MINS, plus cooling
COOK 1 HR

120g (4oz) **wholemeal flour**
100g (3½oz) **walnuts**
85g (3oz) **brown sugar**
2½ tsp **ground cinnamon**
4 tbsp chilled **plant-based butter**,
   cut into small cubes
packet of bought **vegan**
   shortcrust pastry, or **vegan**
   prepared pastry case
170g (6oz) **granulated sugar**
1 tbsp **instant tapioca**, such
   as Minute Tapioca
7 **apples**, such as Granny Smith,
   about 900g (2lb) in total, peeled,
   cored, and thinly sliced
juice of 1 **lemon**

1 Preheat the oven to 180°C (350°F/Gas 4). In a food processor fitted with a metal blade, pulse together the wholemeal flour, walnuts, brown sugar, and ½ teaspoon of the cinnamon to combine. Add the plant-based butter and pulse until the mixture resembles coarse crumbs. Set this streusel topping aside.

2 Roll the pastry for the bottom crust into a 33cm (13in) circle and transfer to a deep 25cm (10in) pie dish. You'll have a 2.5cm (1in) overhang; fold up the overhanging dough, pinch into a rim, and use your fingers to crimp the crust. Refrigerate the pastry case while you make the filling.

3 In a large bowl, whisk together the remaining cinnamon, granulated sugar, and instant tapioca. Add the sliced apples and lemon juice, and toss well to combine. Pour the apple mixture into the prepared pastry case.

4 Using your hands, pick up small handfuls of the streusel topping, press into large crumbs, and break into smaller crumbs as you sprinkle it over the apple filling. Continue, covering the top of the pie evenly, until all the streusel has been used.

5 Put the pie dish on a baking sheet and bake in the lower third of the oven for about 1 hour or until the streusel topping is golden and the filling is bubbling. Check the pie once or twice during baking, and place a piece of foil over the top if the streusel starts to become too brown. Cool the pie at room temperature for 3 hours before slicing.

the good stuff

Walnuts are a good source of the essential fatty acid omega 3, which has benefits for brain health and function. They also contain vital iron for vegans, as well as selenium, zinc, vitamin E, and some B vitamins.

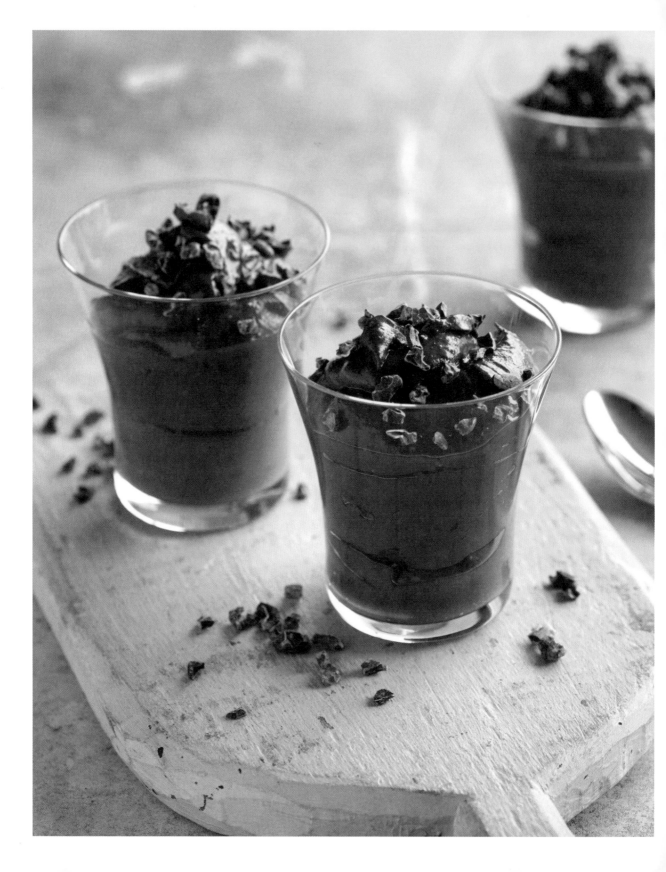

FEELGOOD CHOCOLATE MOUSSE
with cacao & avocados

SERVES 4
PREP 5 MINS, plus chilling

5 ripe **avocados**, about 400g (14oz),
   roughly chopped
30g (1oz) **raw cacao powder**
4 tbsp **maple syrup**
1 tsp **vanilla extract**
4 tbsp **almond** or **coconut milk**
cacao nibs, to serve

1 To make the mousse, place all the ingredients, except the cacao nibs, into a food processor and process them until completely smooth, adding a little extra almond or coconut milk if necessary.

2 Pour the mixture into a serving dish or individual 150ml (5fl oz) glasses. Refrigerate for at least 1 hour, until chilled. To serve, sprinkle the mousse with cacao nibs.

VARIATION

Try stirring through the zest of 1 orange or a teaspoon of strong filtered coffee. You could also top with finely chopped fresh mango, chopped pistachio nuts, or pomegranate seeds.

the good stuff

These little pots have all the richness of a decadent mousse but without the cream, butter, and processed sugar. Raw cacao contains up to four times more antioxidants than regular cocoa powder.

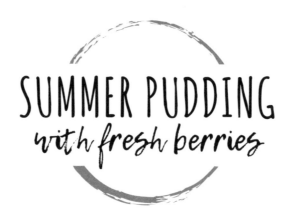

SUMMER PUDDING
with fresh berries

SERVES 6
PREP 15 MINS, plus chilling
COOK 3–4 MINS

900g (2lb) **mixed soft fruits**,
   such as **raspberries**,
   strawberries, blackberries,
   pitted cherries,
   or **blueberries**
50g (1¾oz) **fructose** (fruit sugar)
8–10 thick slices of day-old
   white bread
15g (½oz) **redcurrants**, to decorate
15g (½oz) **mint leaves**, to decorate

1 Place the fruit in a saucepan with the fructose and 3 tablespoons of water. Heat gently and cook for 3–4 minutes or until the juices begin to run from the fruit. Set aside to cool.

2 Remove the crusts from the bread. Cut a circle from 1 slice of bread to fit the bottom of a 1.5 litre (2¾ pint) pudding basin. Arrange the remaining bread, apart from 2 slices, around the sides of the basin, overlapping slightly and leaving no gaps. Place the circle of bread over the gap at the bottom of the basin.

3 Spoon the fruit mixture, together with enough juice to moisten the bread, into the basin. Reserve the remaining juice. Seal in the fruit with a final layer of the remaining bread, trimming to fit as necessary.

4 Cover the pudding with a saucer or small plate and place a heavy weight on top. Place the pudding in the refrigerator for several hours, preferably overnight.

5 To serve, remove the weight and the saucer, and invert the pudding onto a large serving plate. Hold the two together and shake firmly, then carefully remove the pudding basin. Spoon the reserved juice over the pudding and decorate with the redcurrants and mint.

the good stuff

Strawberries are a great option here, as these little berries are even higher in vitamin C than oranges and blackberries. They are also a good source of vitamin K.

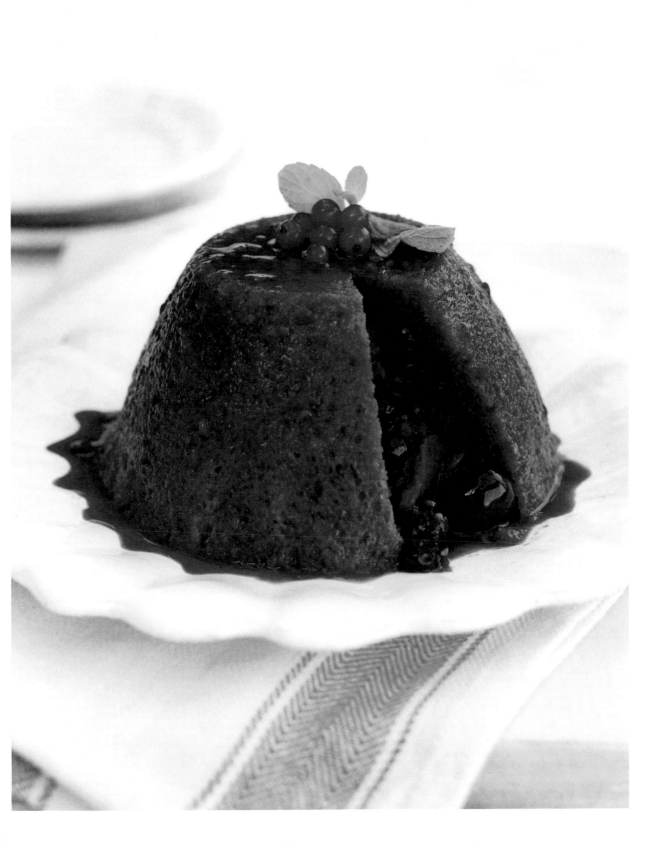

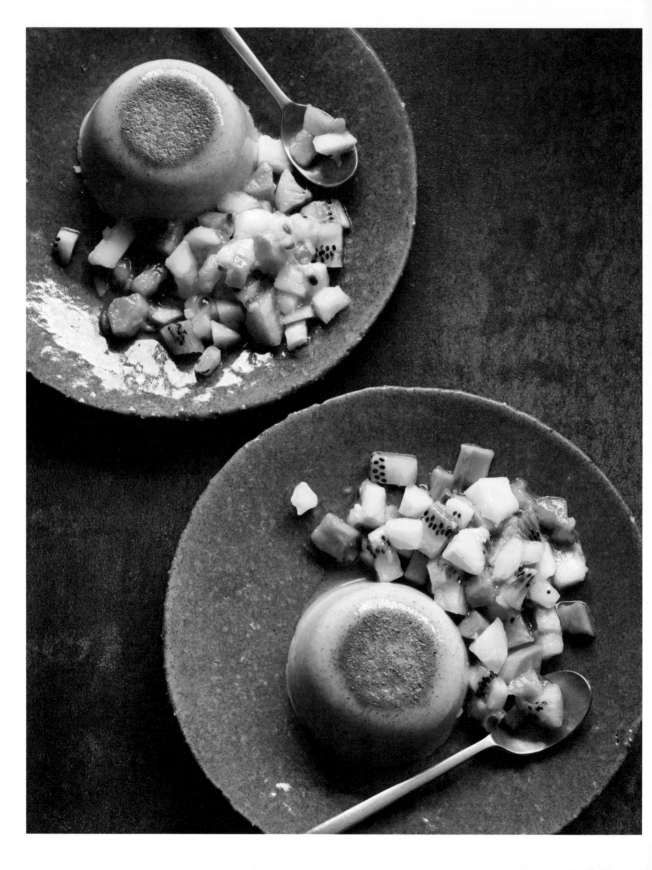

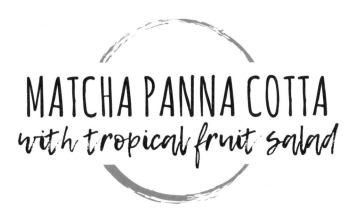

MATCHA PANNA COTTA
with tropical fruit salad

SERVES 4
PREP 25 MINS, plus cooling
  and chilling
COOK 10 MINS

600ml (1 pint) **coconut milk**
6.5g (⅕oz) packet of **vegetarian**
  powdered setting agent
2 tbsp **light soft brown sugar**
½ tsp **matcha powder**
1 tbsp **sunflower oil**

FRUIT SALAD
1 **passion fruit**
½ **ripe mango**, peeled
  and finely diced
1 **ripe kiwi**, finely diced
½ **ripe papaya**, peeled
  and finely diced

1 Transfer 3 tablespoons of the coconut milk into a medium
  heatproof bowl. Scatter the setting agent over the surface of the
milk and whisk it in well, then leave to rest for 5 minutes. Meanwhile,
heat the remaining coconut milk in a small, heavy-based saucepan
over a low heat until it is hot, but not boiling.

2 When the coconut milk is hot, remove it from the heat and pour
  it over the setting agent mixture, whisking well to ensure that all
the powder has dissolved. Whisk in the sugar and matcha powder
until completely combined.

3 Rub the insides of four 150ml (5fl oz) ramekins with a piece of
  kitchen paper dipped in the sunflower oil. Divide the coconut
mixture among the ramekins and allow the mixture to cool before
transferring to the fridge for at least 4–6 hours, until set.

4 To make the fruit salad, cut the passion fruit in half and scrape the
  seeds out into a bowl. Mix the diced fruit with the passion fruit
seeds and set aside.

5 To serve the panna cottas, fill a bowl with hot water and carefully
  dip the outside of each ramekin briefly into the water to loosen the
panna cotta, being careful not to allow the water to drip onto the set
cream. Run a small knife around the edge of the panna cotta and turn
out onto individual serving plates. Serve with the fruit salad.

the good stuff

This dairy-free panna cotta is flavoured with
matcha powder, which contains an amino
acid called theanine that may help to keep
you mentally alert. Mango, kiwi, and papaya
provide antioxidants and natural sweetness.

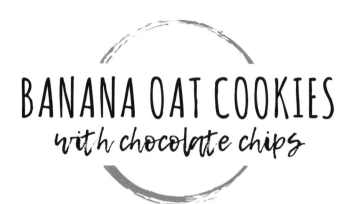

BANANA OAT COOKIES
with chocolate chips

MAKES 16
PREP 15 MINS
COOK 12–14 MINS

1 medium very ripe
   banana, peeled
75g (2½oz) **granulated sugar**
60g (2oz) **brown sugar**
80ml (2½fl oz) **grapeseed oil**
1 tsp **vanilla extract**
125g (4½oz) **plain flour**
170g (6oz) **rolled oats**
½ tsp **bicarbonate of soda**
½ tsp **ground cinnamon**
¼ tsp **sea salt**
85g (3oz) **vegan dark
   chocolate chips**
4 tbsp **unsweetened
   dried coconut**

1 Preheat the oven to 180°C (350°F/Gas 4). Line 2 baking sheets with baking parchment.

2 In a medium bowl, mash the banana with the sugars, grapeseed oil, and vanilla extract until smooth.

3 Stir the flour, rolled oats, bicarbonate of soda, cinnamon, salt, dark chocolate chips, and coconut into the banana mixture, using your hands to ensure the mixture is well combined. It will be very thick.

4 Scoop 3.75cm (1½in) balls of dough onto the baking sheets, spacing them about 6cm (2½in) apart. Using wet hands, gently pat down the cookies into 5cm (2in) rounds. Some chocolate chips might separate from the mixture, if they do, just pat them back into the cookies.

5 Bake for 12–14 minutes or until the cookies are golden. Cool for 3 minutes on the baking sheets, then transfer to a wire rack to cool completely. The cookies will keep in an airtight container for up to 5 days (if they last that long!)

the good stuff

Oats are a real super grain, they contain beta-glucans, a soluble fibre that slows down the absorption of carbs into the bloodstream, which discourages our bodies from making and storing fat.

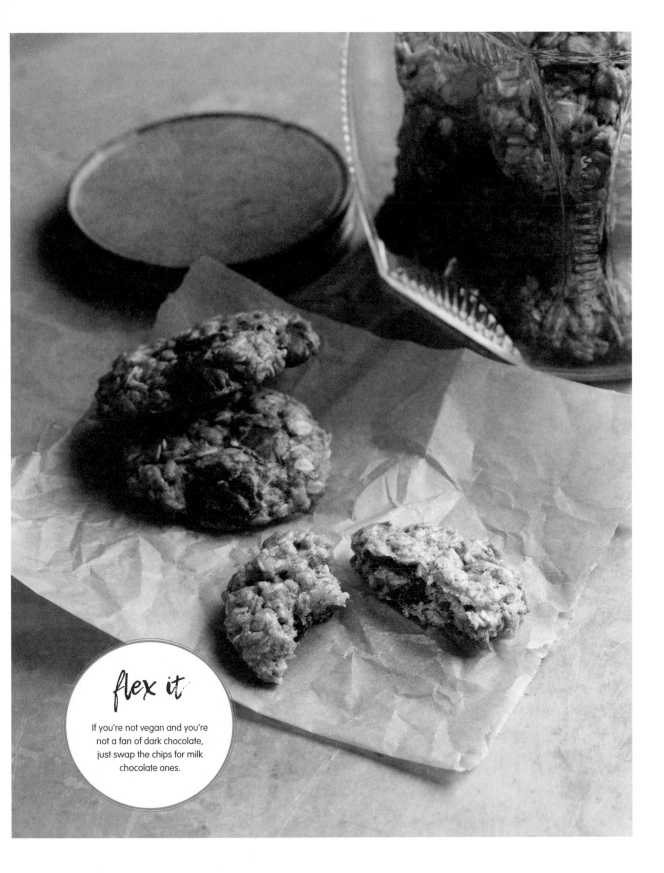

flex it

If you're not vegan and you're
not a fan of dark chocolate,
just swap the chips for milk
chocolate ones.

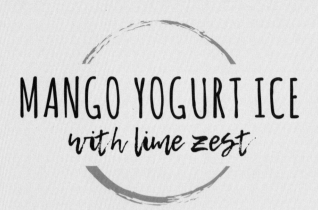

MANGO YOGURT ICE
with lime zest

SERVES 4
PREP 5 MINS, plus cooling
and freezing
COOK 2 MINS

3 ripe **mangoes**, about
225g (8oz) each
125g (4½oz) **caster sugar**
zest and juice of 1 **lime**
4 tbsp **plant-based yogurt**

1 Extract as much fruit as you can from the mangoes, using a knife to scrape the pulp from the skin and stone. Discard the skin and stone and place the pulp in a measuring jug. You should have around 400ml (14fl oz).

2 In a small saucepan, gently heat the sugar and 120ml (4fl oz) of water, and stir until the sugar is dissolved (about 2 minutes). Cool to room temperature. This makes around 200ml (7fl oz) of syrup.

3 In a food processor, blend together the mango pulp, syrup, lime zest and juice, and the yogurt.

4 Place in an ice-cream maker and churn and freeze according to the manufacturer's instructions. Before serving, remove from the freezer and put in the fridge for 20 minutes to soften.

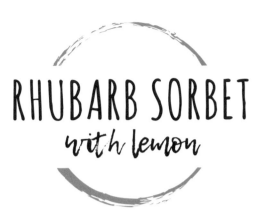

RHUBARB SORBET
with lemon

SERVES 6
PREP 20 MINS, plus
  cooling and freezing
COOK 10 MINS

juice of 1 large **lemon**
140g (5oz) **caster sugar**
450g (1lb) **rhubarb**,
  chopped into 2.5cm
  (1in) pieces
2 tbsp **glucose syrup**

1 Place 225ml (8fl oz) of water, the lemon juice, and caster sugar in a saucepan. Over a low heat, stir until the sugar dissolves.

2 Add the rhubarb, bring to the boil, and simmer for 8 minutes or until the rhubarb is pulpy. Cool to room temperature.

3 Transfer the mixture to a food processor and purée until completely smooth. Stir in the glucose syrup, pulsing briefly for about 25 seconds.

4 Place in an ice-cream maker and churn and freeze according to the manufacturer's instructions. Remove from the freezer 10 minutes before serving.

the good stuff

Eating rhubarb is good for your wellbeing. Vegans don't naturally have as much calcium in their diets as those who eat dairy, but rhubarb provides a good supply of this essential nutrient to promote strong bones and teeth.

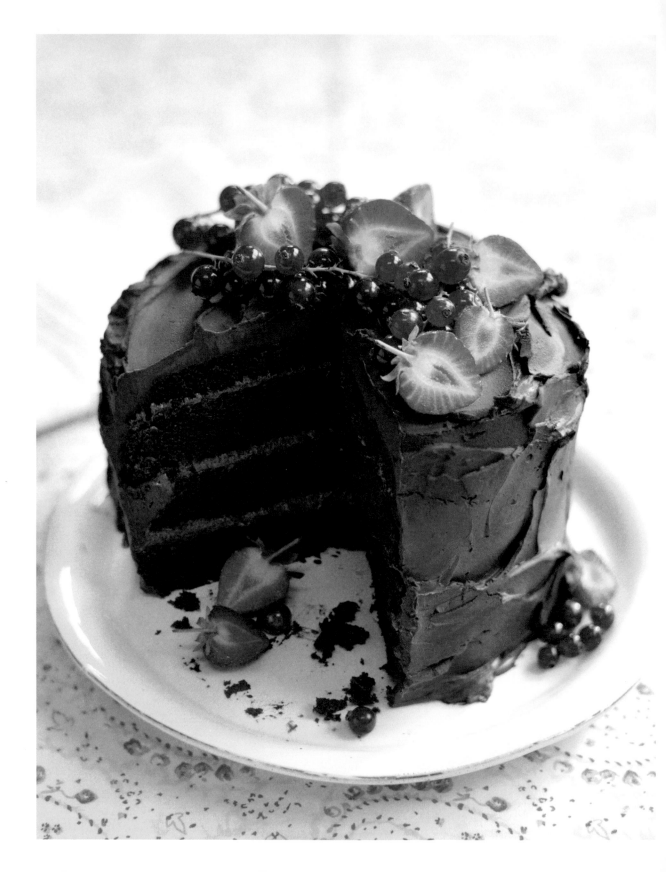

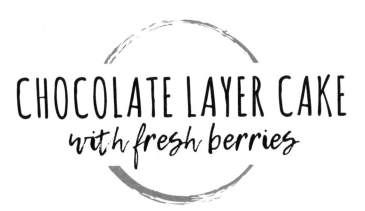

CHOCOLATE LAYER CAKE
with fresh berries

SERVES 10
PREP 30 MINS
COOK 40 MINS, plus cooling

340g (12oz) **plain flour**
400g (14oz) **caster sugar**
1¾ tsp **bicarbonate of soda**
55g (2oz) **vegan cocoa powder**
¼ tsp **salt**
450ml (15fl oz) **unsweetened soya milk** or **water**
100ml (3½fl oz) **corn** or **vegetable oil**, plus extra for greasing
1½ tbsp **white vinegar**
1½ tsp **vanilla extract**

GANACHE
300g (10oz) **vegan dark chocolate**
300ml (10fl oz) **plant-based milk**

TO DECORATE
45g (1½oz) **vegan chocolate**, shaved with a potato peeler, or a selection of **fresh berries**, if preferred

1 Preheat the oven to 180°C (350°F/Gas 4). Grease and line with baking parchment the bases of 2 deep 20cm (8in), round sandwich tins.

2 Sift together into a large bowl the flour, sugar, bicarbonate of soda, cocoa, and salt. In a separate bowl, mix together the liquid ingredients: the soya milk or water, corn oil, vinegar, and vanilla extract, and add to the flour mixture. Stir until smooth.

3 Divide the mixture between the prepared tins, and use a palette knife or spatula to spread evenly. Bake in the oven for about 40 minutes, until risen and firm to the touch.

4 Cool in the tins for 10 minutes then turn out onto a wire rack, remove the baking parchment and leave to cool completely. Slice each cake in half horizontally.

5 To make the ganache, melt the dark chocolate and combine with the plant-based milk.

6 Sandwich the cakes together using half the ganache for the first 3 layers. Spread the remainder on the top and sides and rough up with a knife. Sprinkle with chocolate shavings or decorate with fresh berries, if you like.

POMEGRANATE & RASPBERRY GRANITA
with fresh mint

SERVES 8
PREP 20 MINS, plus freezing

1kg (2¼lb) **seedless watermelon**
  (about 1½ mini watermelons)
  or ½ large watermelon, skinned
  and diced
175g (6oz) **raspberries**,
  plus extra to decorate
150g (5½oz) **pomegranate seeds**,
  plus extra to decorate
large handful of **mint leaves**,
  plus extra to decorate
1–2 tbsp **maple syrup**

1 Place half the watermelon in a blender or food processor, along
  with half the raspberries, pomegranate seeds, and mint leaves.
Process to a liquid and pour into a large bowl. Blend the remaining
watermelon, raspberries, pomegranate seeds, and mint, and combine
with the first batch of liquid. (Working in batches prevents the blender
or food processor overflowing.)

2 Put the resulting liquid through a fine metal sieve and strain into a
  large bowl, pressing down with the back of a spoon to extract all
the liquid from the pulp. Discard the pulp. If you are using seeded
watermelon, also discard any fragments of seed.

3 Whisk in the maple syrup as needed, depending on the sweetness
  of the watermelon. Remember that the sweetness will be dulled on
freezing, so adjust according to your taste.

4 Tip the liquid into a large, freezerproof airtight container and
  freeze. Remove from the freezer every 2 hours and use a metal fork
to scrape the frozen sides back into the granita, crushing the resulting
crystals as you go. Repeat three times, until it is completely frozen.

5 Remove from the freezer and put in the fridge for 30 minutes
  before serving. To serve, scrape out layers of crystals into
individual serving bowls or glasses
and garnish with extra raspberries,
pomegranate seeds,
and mint leaves.

the good stuff

This fresh-tasting granita is a simple superfood
and dairy-free alternative to ice cream, and
doesn't require an ice-cream maker. It's packed
with antioxidant pomegranates, vitamin C-rich
raspberries, and immune-boosting mint.

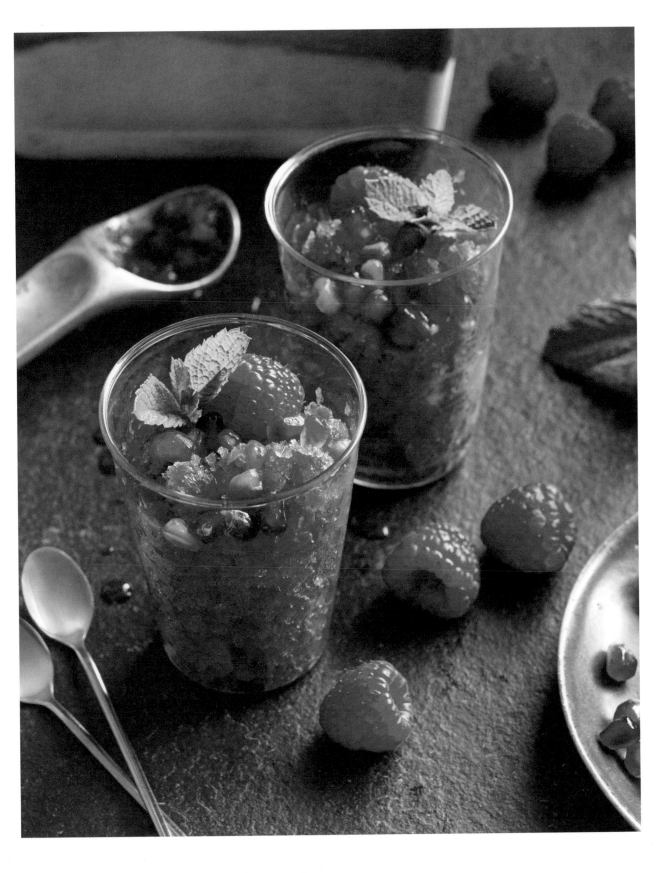

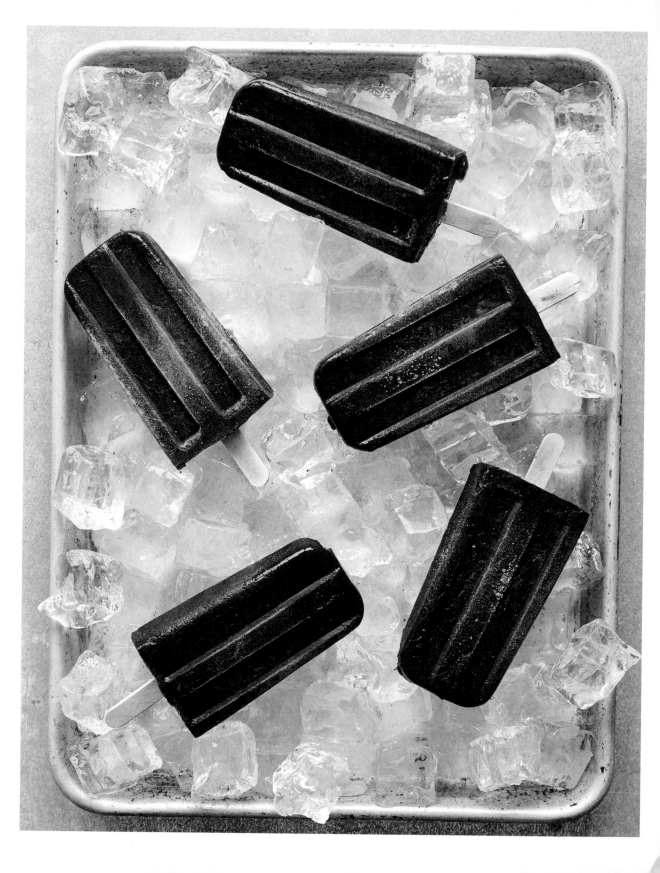

BERRY & LIME MUNG BEAN ICE POPS
with sweet agave nectar

MAKES 10
PREP 20 MINS, plus freezing

225g (8oz) **blueberries**
225g (8oz) **blackberries**
60g (2oz) cooked **mung beans**
3 tbsp **lime juice**
80ml (2½fl oz) **agave nectar**

1 In a blender or food processor, purée the blueberries, blackberries, mung beans, lime juice, agave, and 80ml (2½fl oz) of water until completely smooth.

2 Pour the mixture through a fine sieve to remove the seeds. Press the mixture against the sieve to retain as much liquid as possible.

3 Pour the liquid into 10 lollipop moulds. Insert a stick into each mould. Freeze for at least 6 hours or overnight before serving.

VARIATION

For a flavour variation, swap the berries for raspberries and strawberries. For a taste of the tropics, use fresh pineapple and mango.

the good stuff

These make the perfect low-calorie treat. Mung beans are packed with vitamin B6, which supports adrenal function, and helps to calm and maintain a healthy nervous system. Agave nectar is a great vegan alternative to honey.

INDEX

Storecupboard ingredients in the recipes such as flour or flavourings are not included in this index. Herbs or spices in large amounts are included.

ACKNOWLEDGMENTS

Material in this publication was first published in Great Britain in *Allergy-Free Cookbook* (2007), *The Cooking Book* (2008), *The Diabetes Cookbook* (2010), *The More Veg Cookbook* (2013), *Mediterranean Cookbook* (2014), *Grains as Mains* (2015), *Plant Based Cookbook* (2016), *Superfood Breakfasts* (2016), *Power Bowls* (2016), *Energy Bites* (2016), *Power Pulses* (2017), *Super Clean Super Foods* (2017), *100 Weight Loss Bowls* (2017), *Sprouted* (2017).

All photography and artworks © Dorling Kindersley

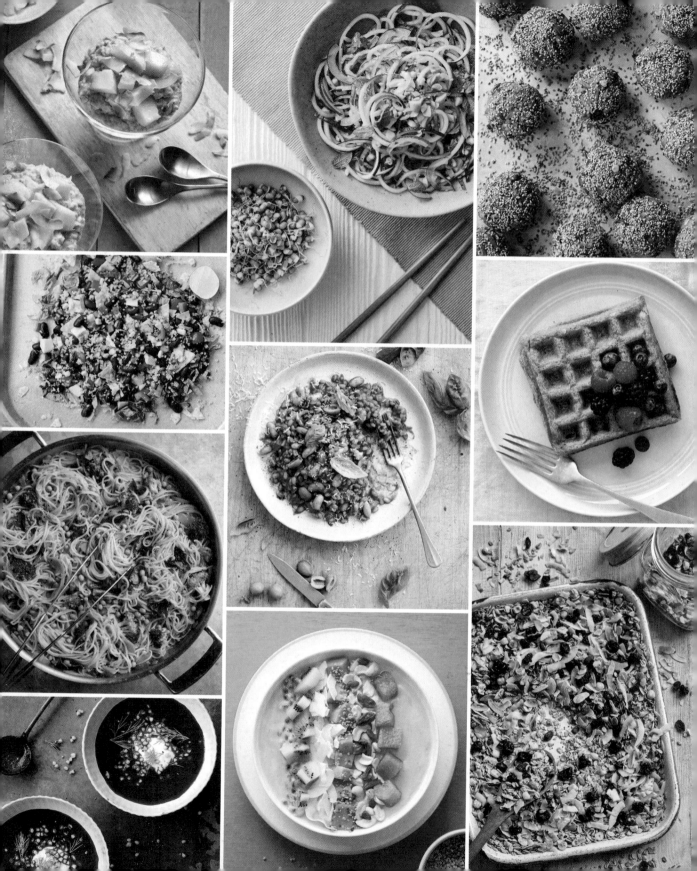